Stress in Theatre Nursing

13
pg. 37
41
23

To the memory of my father

Norman Frederick Astbury, CBE

whose particular interest in this study inspired
him to provide the following appropriate
quotation:

'Ut tensio sic vis'

(Robert Hooke, 1678)

Stress in Theatre Nursing

Charmian Astbury

RSCN, SRN, BA, MSc

This study was submitted as a research thesis to
the University of Manchester in part fulfilment of
the requirement for the degree of Master of
Science in the Faculty of Medicine.

ROYAL COLLEGE OF NURSING
RESEARCH SERIES

Scutari Press

Aims of the Series

To encourage the appreciation and dissemination of nursing research by making relevent studies of high quality available to the profession at reasonable cost.

The RCN is happy to publish this series of research reports. The projects were chosen by the individual research worker and the findings are those of the researcher and relate to the particular subject in the situation in which it was studied. The RCN in accordance with its policy of promoting research awareness among members of the profession commends this series for study but views expressed do not necessarily reflect RCN policy.

Scutari Press

Viking House, 17–19 Peterborough Road,
Harrow, Middlesex HA1 2AX, England

A subsiduary of Scutari Projects, the publishing company of
the Royal College of Nursing

First published 1988

British Library Cataloguing in Publication Data:

Astbury, Charmian
    Stress in theatre nursing
    1. Nurses. Stress
    I. Title II. Series
    610.73'01'9

    ISBN 1 871364 01 9

Typeset by Action Typesetting Ltd., Gloucester
Printed and bound in Great Britain by Billing & Sons, Worcester

Contents

1 Introduction and summary

There is a considerable body of work and an equally formidable array of anecdotes within the world of nursing suggesting that working in an operating theatre is stressful. Not only is there a direct relationship between stress, low morale and poor recovery rates in patients (Revans, 1972), but there is also recognised difficulty in the recruitment and retention of nursing staff in areas perceived as stressful. This present research study sought as a first step towards a solution for this depressing situation to identify within the work environment of operating theatres and their support wards:

- those experiences perceived as stressful by nurses;
- whether or not controllable elements in the experience of stress could be established;
- whether or not a relationship existed between the stress and satisfaction experiences of the day;
- whether the experiences of the nurses in the theatre influenced the experience of the nurses in the ward.

The design parameters of this study were:

1. the operating theatres of five different health authorities were used in the study in order to minimise possible observer bias;
2. routine operating sessions only were observed;
3. sessions providing the data were classified as 'morning', 'afternoon' or 'all day';
4. the five-day period from Monday to Friday was 'the week';
5. one week's pilot study was planned in one health authority;
6. the full exploratory study was planned to take place over four weeks in four other different health authorities (H1, H2, H3 and H4).

1

The observation and interview methods used in this study were designed to record both quantifiable data items (such as observations detailing number and type of operation, time taken and so forth) and qualitative data (comments about the wholly subjective and individual experience of the nurse concerned). As many experiences were only mildly troublesome ('they might have told me the electrician was coming') or mildly agreeable ('this has been a pleasant day'), the number of experiences as well as the intensity of the nurse's perception of them would be recorded. The intensity of experience was identified by the use of a rating scale.

Thus, not only were the actual number of stressful and satisfactory experiences or incidents recorded but also an indication of the quality of the experience. The results of recording the number of experiences demonstrated that the number of satisfactory occurrences in the nurse's day outweighed the stressful ones by about two to one. However, in spite of this favourable statement, once the scores for both stress and satisfaction experiences obtained by using the rating scale were taken into account, the results of this study appeared to suggest that the perception of intensity of stress is such that its experience constitutes an influential, and probably major, element in the day. Figure 1 uses the mean rank scores for satisfaction and stress experienced in the wards and theatres to demonstrate the pressure of stress and its influence on satisfaction. In three of the four hospitals, stress tended to be the more prominent experience and in H2 (which did have acknowledged difficulties in both wards and theatres) satisfaction scores were much lower than in the other hospitals and its stress levels were correspondingly high. H2, in fact, produced the highest stress levels in this study. H1, which was the hospital in which I had enjoyed my first sister's post many years ago, was still a marvellous place in which to work, and it was very exciting to see my personal impressions mirrored in these results.

H1 managed its time better than any other hospital in the study, for the overrun/underrun time of the routine lists observed was modest. H2, on the other hand, overran and underran on routine lists to the extent that half of the routine lists overran by four hours and in so doing doubled the routine planned four-hour session time. (Their underrun time did not compensate for this in any way.) H3 had the worst underrun times in the study and this appeared to be directly linked to beds being 'blocked' on the wards. H4 acknowledged that the break between sessions was being used to absorb

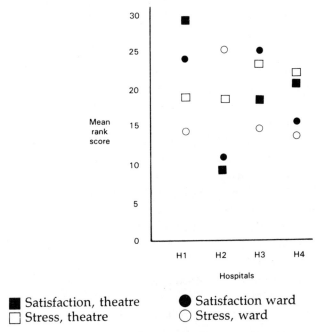

■ Satisfaction, theatre   ● Satisfaction ward
□ Stress, theatre   ○ Stress, ward

Figure 1 Comparison of mean rank scores for stress and satisfaction in theatres and wards, by hospital

the time demands made on their routine sessions.

In this study eight significant stress relationships were identified, one of which related to patient care and was an appropriate and proper experience within the acute environment of the operating theatre. The other seven significant stresses, which included the overrun/underrun time, should, it could reasonably be argued, not be present at all for these were either organisational, environmental or man-management stresses. It is suggested, with caution as this is a first study in this area, that these statistically significant stress results indicate the presence of poor communication (shown by list inaccuracies), a lack of common organisational purpose (the overrun/underrun time), weak day-to-day organisation (meal-break difficulties), poor understanding of work environment (lack of windows) and weak man-management (skill-mix difficulties, observed stress, temperature perceived as 'hot'). Such matters are not unique to health care. They may be found as areas of stress in any human organisation. All those involved in the working of the stressed organisation should be encouraged to tackle their particular problems and difficulties.

There is nothing new or surprising in the findings of this present study except, sadly, to discover that the problems continue. Both the Lewin Report of the late 1970s (Lewin, 1978) and the work of Revans earlier in that decade stated that the solutions to the problems in operating theatres and wards can only be found in those operating theatres and wards.

The first section of this study considers a review of the available literature and describes the theoretical background to the study which includes both general and specific aspects of stress, working relationships in the theatre and associated conflict areas, as well as functional aspects of the day-to-day management.

The research proper follows in the next section and the analysis, discussion of the significant results and tentative conclusions are to be found in the third. The bibliography lists work that ranges from the opinions and comments expressed in the nursing and medical journals to sound research theses, reports and government documents. In addition there are six appendixes in which certain aspects of the study are recorded in greater detail. Appendix V includes a selection of anecdotal comments indicating the wider work perspective of routine operating sessions and the pressures of the day.

Part 1: Literature review and theoretical background

2 Parameters, Background and Definitions

This study was an attempt to discover whether or not stress is experienced by qualified nurses working in operating theatres and those in the relevant supporting wards who have the care of patients on their day of operation. One main hypothesis was that theatre and ward nursing staff, aware of the potential for danger to the patient, experience stress should a change occur in the expected organisation of the operating day. A further hypothesis which could be of significance in relation to postoperative recovery rates (Revans, 1964) was that stress experienced by nurses in the operating theatres could well be reflected in the stress experienced by the nurses working in the relevant wards. A number of possible stress-producing factors associated with the work of the operating theatre were examined, such as the number of learner nurses present, the seniority of the staff in charge, use of operating session time, and presence or absence of windows. The study variables are listed in tables 1 and 2, chapter 9, and in appendix IV.

Because of the limitations of time the study was planned as a pilot study, that is, a compact, limited fact-finding study to establish some baseline information for further work in the field of nursing staff stress and the work organisation of operating days. The sample was small: a selection of hospitals in five different area health authorities only was used, one to test the methods and four for the main study. The information collected was confined to that which concerned the working of routine planned operating sessions.

The need for the construction of a valid research tool is discussed by Clark and Hockey (1979) and other nurse research authors, such as Polit and Hungler (1978) and Treece and Treece (1977). In this study the first hospital provided the information required for the construction of the research tool (see appendix III), the others being used for the data collection of the main study. It was hoped that, by selecting hospitals in different area health authorities, the information so collected for the study would not only reflect current practice but also minimise possible observer bias.

STUDY BACKGROUND

It has been recognised for some years that hospitals are anxiety-producing, stressful organisations (Menzies, 1970; Revans, 1964, 1972, 1976). Stress and anxiety is experienced not only by patients and their relatives but also by the medical and nursing staff who have the responsibility for the cure and care of the patients. Studies in this present decade by Leatt and Schneck (1980) and Hingley et al (1986) suggest that stress, although it may differ in type, is experienced throughout the whole of hospital organisation. Other work though, such as that of Hay and Oken (1972), sees certain areas within the hospital, for instance intensive care units and operating theatres, as being of particular stress to nursing staff. Many of the stresses and strains experienced in the operating theatre are not recognised consciously by the individual as they are associated with the unconscious fears aroused by surgical assault on, and exposure to, the living, helpless, diseased or injured body. These fears may be internalised, coped with and distanced by the defence mechanisms of the individual concerned (Menzies, 1970; Lazarus, 1964; Janis, 1958). These contained stresses contribute to what has been described as the 'combat' exhaustion of those who work in high emotional risk areas (Hay and Oken, 1972; Holesclaw, 1965) and to the irrational responses to minor irritations that can be exhibited by those who work in such areas (Coleman, 1978). Work by Nichols, Springford and Searle (1981), though, suggests that the stress situation in what are regarded as high emotional risk areas may not be as negative as some authorities would appear to indicate, and that the psychosocial conditions within which nursing staff work are as powerful determinants of happiness as the type of nursing pursued.

The complexity of work in the operating department has increased. New technologies, new drugs, new materials and techniques have contributed to the ever-expanding scope of the service available to the patient. The skills and competencies of the staff involved have had to keep pace with all advances, and obsolescence of knowledge can be a very real problem (Tobin, 1974; Toffler, 1970).

The changing nature of care imposes stresses and strains on the nurse (The Committee on Nursing, 1972), something that stronger organisation of nursing could help to contain (Kinston, 1987). Nurses who are confident and secure within their professional roles are able to acknowledge the presence of stress and find solutions (Revans, 1976), a particularly important ability in the individual whom it is hoped to recruit and retain in a work area known to have difficulties in attracting staff (National Audit Office, 1987). Defence mechanisms may well be the last resort for many nurses and stress will be internalised and contained (Menzies, 1970; Lazarus, 1964) leading eventually to poor quality patient care.

The present study was designed to identify causes of stress, particularly those in the work environment, and the organisational elements amenable to control or improvement by better understanding of the operating day in both theatre and wards (Robson, 1986; Peters and Waterman, 1982). There was no attempt made to measure physiological stresses, for instance recording the pulse rate, palmar sweat index or hormone excretion levels, techniques which have been used with success in studies of patient experience of stress (Boore, 1978; Munday, 1973), although further work could make use of such techniques to establish the physiological levels of stress in staff who admit to stress. This present study was concerned to record certain background information as well as the subjective individual comments of the nurse working within one particular environment at one particular time. The perception of the individual concerned as to what was viewed as stressful, as well as that particular individual's ability to resolve or ignore the situation, was taken into account.

That there are common elements that cause anxiety within the organisation of the operating day is recognised in the number and variety of existing articles, the subject matter of which ranges from optimum temperature (Lamont, 1977) to working relationships with consultants (Coghill et al, 1970). Both the Briggs (The Committee on Nursing, 1972) and Lewin (Department of Health and Social Security, 1970) Reports comment on significant causes for concern in the organisation of the operating day including problems associated with the operating list.

The function of the operating list is to control the organisation of both the ward and the theatre and includes medical, nursing and ancillary staff on operating days. Preoperative preparation, patient fasting and premedication, the transport of patients, the planning of X-ray time, etc., all depend for their optimum results on adherence to the schedule. The preparation of instruments and equipment, carrying out of safety and checking procedures, and the reception, recovery and return of the patients are planned for in accordance with the information on the list (Campbell, 1979; Matthias, 1973). That changes do occur and that they are dangerous and sometimes unavoidable are acknowledged in the Joint Memorandum of the Medical Defence Union and the Royal College of Nursing (1978) in the following extracts:

1.4   Mistakes occur when changes are made on theatre lists...

2.9   Any alteration to the operating list must be made on every relevant copy by a designated person.

References to the significance of co-operation between nursing and medical staff in the compilation of operating lists are to be found in the Briggs and Lewin Reports. Numerous nursing articles published (Phillips, 1980; Campbell, 1979; Hulme, 1973; Revans, 1972; Hassell, 1971) as well as many individual unpublished surveys (Duffey and Worthington, 1980) refer to the problems associated with operating list change. General observation in almost any operating theatre and appropriate ward will confirm that changes do occur and that the nursing staff involved appear to experience increasing pressure and high levels of stress as a result. Patients also suffer stress and, although their experience is outside the framework of this study, it is perhaps appropriate to mention that one patient in this study had to return home following, in his view, too many alterations to the list order.

STUDY DEFINITIONS

Some of the more significant terms in the present study are used with the following meanings.

Nursing staff

Nurse: Any member of the qualified nursing staff, on the roll or on the register, male or female, and of any grade. There is a further categorisation for the purposes of analysis into theatre-experienced qualified staff and qualified staff.

Nursing auxiliary: Assistant to the nursing staff without formal qualifications but with experience of work in the operating theatre.

Learners/learner nurses: Any student or pupil nurse in training.

Work environment

The definitions of the terms under this heading are based on the recommendations of the Lewin Report.

Operating department: An operating department is a unit consisting of one or more operating suites together with ancillary accommodation provided for the common use of those suites, such as changing rooms, rest rooms, reception, transfer and recovery areas and circulation space.

Operating suite: An operating suite comprises the operating theatre together with its own ancillary areas, namely, anaesthetic room, a room for setting up instrument trolleys, a disposal room, a scrub-up and gowning area and an exit area which may be part of the circulation space of the operating department.

Operating theatre: An operating theatre is the room in which surgical operations and certain diagnostic procedures are carried out.

Operating list: The operating list is the work schedule compiled by the medical staff in consultation with the nursing staff which can reasonably be expected to be completed by the surgical teams within a defined session. The recommendations of the Lewin Report include that the list should be typed for distribution and contain the following information, without the use of abbreviations:

- Name of patient – surname and first name(s)
- Age
- Sex
- Registered hospital or unit number
- Nature, site and side of operation
- Ward
- Date and time of operation
- Name of consultant surgeon
- Name of consultant anaesthetist
- Any special requirements or considerations

Operating session: The operating session is the time allowed for each scheduled list of operations to be performed, usually 3½–4 hours in the morning or afternoon, and sometimes arranged as an all-day session.

Stress

The Shorter Oxford Dictionary definitions of stress include:

1. To subject (a person) to force or compulsion, to constraint or restraint.
2. To subject to hardship, to afflict, to harass, to oppress.
3. To subject (a bodily organ, a mental faculty) to strain, to over-work, to fatigue.

Other definitions of stress suggest that it is:

1. The non-specific response of the body to any demand, whether physical, psychological, physiological or socio-cultural (Selye, 1978).
2. An important intervention between an individual and his environment (Gatley, 1981).
3. The unresolved ability to regain the capacity to adjust to an imposed situation (Pollitt, 1977).

Stress is frequently defined in engineering terms (Wallace, 1978) and such words as 'tension', 'strain' and 'breaking point' are familiar in this context.

The most useful of the many descriptions of the stress concept in terms of what is required for this present study is felt to be that of the watch-spring analogy. A certain amount of tension is required to make a watch-spring function but, should the watch be overwound, the spring is overstressed, balance is destroyed and function ceases.

3 | General aspects of stress

In this chapter brief consideration is given to some of the general and social stresses that affect both society and nursing. As indicated in chapter 1 there was to be no attempt at a total discussion of stress and its physical, physiological and psychological aspects. The purpose of the present study was to attempt to identify some of the environmental and organisational stresses which might prove to be avoidable within the work situation in hospitals on operating days.

> 'Staying alive and healthy today is like staying alive and healthy in the middle of a war. The ever present enemy kills and maims . . . with stress . . . know your information, plan your defence and spot the casualties.' (Coleman, 1978)

> 'Popularisation of mental health wisdom has communicated the thought, utterly bizarre, in one of the most frightening periods of human history, that the mentally healthy person is free from all anxiety and meets life with radiant confidence.' (White, 1976)

It would appear to be generally acknowledged that the life stresses of modern Western society are of a greater pressure than they ever have been, and are probably increasing. The dominance of stress diseases is one measure of this. A survey undertaken at one major teaching hospital indicated that one in five patients admitted to the medical wards was there because he or she had tried to commit suicide (Coleman, 1978). People within today's society suffer from many conditions exacerbated or produced by excessive stress, and nowadays we are not surprised to know that high blood pressure, cerebral haemorrhage, heart attacks, gastric ulcers, alcoholism, dermatitis, back pain, suicide and the need to smoke may well be stress-related.

However, stress is also a function of the interaction between man and his environment (Pollitt, 1977), forming a normal and vital part

13

of life (Toynbee, 1966; Selye, 1978). White (1976) asks what the transactions are that actually take place between man and his environment for, in actuality, there are many situations that can be met only by compromise or even resignation. He uses the military metaphor, as does Coleman (1978), to describe the process of adapting to stress, using phrases like 'strategic retreat', 'regrouping of forces', 'seeking fresh intelligence' and 'deploying new weapons'. Others define an understanding of stress and strain in engineering terms (Wallace, 1978; Woolstone, 1978). A useful definition which embraces both concepts is that excessive stress may be thought of as an unresolved inability to regain the capacity to adjust to an imposed situation (Pollitt, 1977). Adjustment and adaptation do not mean either the total triumph over the environment or a total surrender to it, but rather a striving towards an acceptable compromise, a balance (Selye, 1978). This is a concept that fits well with the organic nature of management required to cope with the disrupted environment to be found in hospitals (Pembrey, 1980). White (1976) states that adaptation behaviour requires the simultaneous management of at least three variables, which are:

1.   the securing of adequate information;
2.   the maintaining of satisfactory internal conditions;
3.   the individual maintaining some degree of autonomy.

Should there be a failure of any of these components necessary to the function of adaptation, excessive stress will result.

These adaptive measures lie at the heart of the philosophies of good management and the pursuit of excellence (Robson, 1986). Drucker (1967) discusses the importance of the individual's contribution to the organisation which contains aspects of all three measures of adaptation. Job satisfaction, well-being and development of the individual are all vital to the functioning of the organisation and depend on the individual responsibility, contribution and autonomy of the person concerned, at whatever level he may be working (Robson, 1986; Peters and Waterman, 1982; Drucker, 1967; Herzberg, 1966; Maslow, 1943, 1970). Anything blocking these approaches whether attitudinal, organisational or environmental will cause conflict, stress and failure to adapt. Goodman (1978) argues that women in Western society are denied many of the freedoms to develop within an organisation for, he says, they are 'traditionally taught not to complain, not to react aggressively, not to blame others; as a result they frequently withdraw from and internalise their problems'. The ill-advisedness of misconceptions concerning socially-determined gender roles and values that not only do not suit many individuals but are also seen as a source of stress is discussed by Gebhard (1978). The implications of such ideas are of great relevance in a study of stress in nurses on operating days for women are still more numerous than men in the nursing profession (Hockey, 1976).

Although nursing as a stress-producing work activity does not appear to feature in some of the statistical data concerning which jobs in society predispose towards which stress-related conditions (Coleman, 1978), that stress does exist in nursing in general is recognised. Members of the profession themselves have contributed to a growing body of knowledge evident in their discussions concerning particular care areas (Brett, 1978; Melia, 1977). Several major reports produced during the 1970s addressed these concerns and remain as relevant today as they were when first published. Of particular importance to the present study are the following:

- The Tunbridge Report: 'The care of the health of hospital staff' (Great Britain Central Health Services Council and Scottish Health Services Council, 1986)
- The Lewin Report: 'The organisation and staffing of operating theatres' (Department of Health and Social Security, 1970)
- The Briggs Report: 'The report of the Committee on Nursing' (The Committee on Nursing, 1972)

These three reports recognised the presence of stress and the problems caused by stress in the nursing profession.

Tunbridge points out that not only was the National Health Service the largest employer in the country at that time but also that it had to make an intensified use of resources. Twenty years on this still holds true. The information contained in the Tunbridge Report proved so appropriate to a consideration of nursing staff stress that it is difficult to resist quoting it in full. The report states that hospital staff are seen as continually having to adjust to the emotional stress that is aroused when dealing with human beings in states of sickness and anxiety, and that nurses in particular must begin to cope with such influences at a young and impressionable age.

> 'It has been said many times that in every industry manpower is the most expensive item. This is particularly true of the hospital industry which devotes more time training the skills of its employees than is done

in the general run of industry but which uses them . . . without sufficient
regard to their actual physical needs, let alone their emotional ones.'
(Tunbridge Report, Section 134)

Guidelines to assist the introduction of occupational health
services for staff were issued by the Royal College of Nursing
during the same year that the Tunbridge Report was published
(Royal College of Nursing, 1968).

Occupational health service departments are developing within
most hospitals and health authorities now, as are counselling
services for nursing staff (Royal College of Nursing, 1978) although
the RCN working party report investigating the counselling available to nursing staff contains a concluding comment to the effect
that services to support nurses under stress are 'scarce, inadequate,
fragmented and not always known to those in need'. In the report,
'Counselling in Nursing' (Royal College of Nursing, 1978) reference
is made to the indications within the health services of the persis-
tence of the traditional attitude that nurses must always be able to
cope, whatever the circumstances. The pressure of an attitude of
this sort can only be stressful when dealing with the unstable
environment of hospital organisation and the implications appear
to be that managerial support is weak. Wastage of nursing staff may
be understandable but it is undesirable (Annandale-Steiner, 1979)
and to leave the situation is the solution of many nursing staff
(Menzies, 1970; Revans, 1964).

Even such a limited discussion as this on some general aspects of
stress would be incomplete without a reference to the stress of
boredom, a problem more usually associated with the simple and
repetitive jobs of industry. Briggs indicates that boredom can be a
problem within the National Health Service (The Committee on
Nursing, 1972, paragraph 176) and Selye (1978) recognises the
stress of what he describes as 'compulsory inactivity'. Staff
boredom with the activities that have become routine increases
patient anxiety (Nursing Times, 1979) and boredom is seen as one
factor in the failure to achieve adequate communication. Maggs
(1981) discusses historical attitudes that have moulded the nursing
culture of today, including the possible reasons for the still inherent
feeling in nursing staff that it is time-wasting to stop and talk to
patients. This may be a contributory factor in what could be a
vicious circle of staff 'boredom', lack of communication and patient
anxiety. Willingham (1971) mentions boredom, or more accurately
lack of it, in a more positive sense in relation to operating theatres

in his statement that there is always something to keep one interested in theatres. Such statements should perhaps be treated with caution in view of studies exploring the historical reasons for attitudes in nursing (Maggs, 1981) as well as the use of guilt as a nurse control (Hillier, 1980). 'Monotony at work is to be avoided at all cost and this is a problem for management' (Woolstone, 1978).

Staff development, counselling and good management practices should cope with the over- and under-use of staff in acute areas, for human disease and injury are not conditions that produce an even flow of activity. What may contribute to stress even now is a reluctance to admit that empty times do occur. Shame and its consequent guilt are still used as a control in the culture of nursing and this should not occur (Hillier, 1980).

The brief discussion in this chapter of points raised in the available and relevant literature has concentrated upon a small area of the vast complexity that is stress. The aim of this study is to determine whether stress is experienced by nursing staff on operating days and how it is manifested. This consideration of some of the more general aspects of stress provides a modest theoretical background to the study. The next three chapters consider some of the particular stress experiences within one particular group forming one part of the hospital organisation, that is the nurses having the care of the patient on the day of operation. The working relationships of operating theatres, the design of operating theatres, the function of the operating list and, finally, some aspects of nurse–patient relationships are discussed within this perspective.

4 The operating department

'The aim of the theatre team should be to enable the patient to have the operation performed by the surgeon to the best of his ability and in the safest possible surroundings.' (Dixon, 1976)

The hospital is a human work system of recognised complexity and deep anxieties; both are acknowledged causes for concern and research (Revans, 1964, 1972, 1976; Menzies, 1970). An aim as apparently straightforward as the one just quoted is not as easy to achieve as its 'straight-forwardness' implies in such a setting, for the priorities of those co-operating in the aim of safe patient care in the operating theatre may differ.

Such conflict is inevitable within any human work organisation and indeed it is recognised as a necessary element in organisational development (Wallace, 1978). But conflict also produces stress. This chapter will consider some aspects of two possible sources of conflict in the operating department. If the surgeon is to be able to operate 'to the best of his ability and in the safest possible surroundings' (Dixon, 1978), the possibility of conflict must be acknowledged and its effects, if not nullified, at least minimised. As is stated by Revans (1972) 'the critical problems of hospitals are on their wards and in their theatres and they will be solved only on those wards and in those theatres; they will not be solved elsewhere'.

The existence of any institution or organisation implies that there are certain needs within society that require to be met and which can be met only by the collective co-operative activity of members of that society, irrespective of the presence or absence of any particular individual within that organisation or institution (Kogan et al, 1971). The hospital is one such organisation. The wards and departments of a hospital are organisational units inter-relating within the whole, creating a system or set of systems. As Pembrey

19

(1980) indicated, the relationship between an environment and an organisation may be considered by approaching the analysis through the study of systems, and she explores the concept of organic management in relation to the disrupted and unstable environment present in hospitals.

This concept is echoed in the work of those who, like Dixon (1978), consider that the nursing team is the working, decision-making unit in the operating department whose direct liaison with the surgical team is a vital organisational function. The need for functional communication pathways is a prerequisite for the under-standing of any organisation (Revans, 1976). The studies produced by nurses during the 1970s not only indicate that this is realised but also demonstrate that they are aware that structural design can be as influential upon communication pathways as can working relationships (Phillips, 1980; Perry, 1978; Craig, 1978).

The hospital is an organisation that exists for the cure and care of patients. The operating theatre is a unit that contributes to this aim by providing the necessary environment and support in order that the required surgical intervention may take place in safety on the wellness/illness continuum (Hoeller, 1974) of a particular individual. But, for the primary goal of the health care systems to be effective, those who comprise the multidisciplinary teams within the complex structure must have some understanding of the organisational, group and individual needs and how these needs interact (Claus and Bailey, 1977; Robson, 1986). Figure 2 provides a diagrammatic representation of such interactions. The need for some formal understanding of the working of an organisation is found repeatedly in the literature. The theatre environment encompasses a series of interlocking systems which include the functioning of the teams that deliver the surgery (Dudley, 1976) as well as the broader aspects of structural design (Perry, 1978).

The interaction between an individual and the environment is of course an individual experience and the correct stress balance of this interaction is personal (Gatley, 1981; Selye, 1978). Undue stress is to be found in maladaption or failure to adapt to any environment (Pollitt, 1977). Coleman (1978) sees stresses as dividing into three major groups: environmental, social and personal – three useful starting points. This study presents the data within the broad categories of environmental stress, in which there are certain design and administrative elements, and of personal or social stress in which category the individual perception of stress and satisfaction experience was considered.

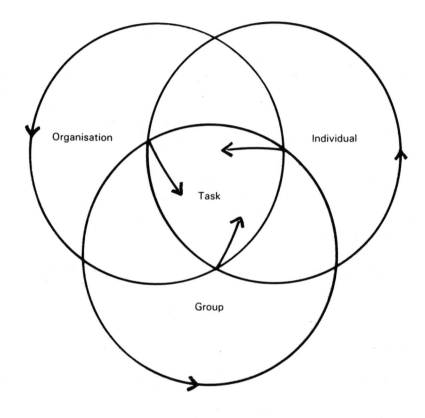

Figure 2 Diagrammatic representation of the overlapping and possible blocking interactions of the organisation, group and individual in relation to the task (after Claus and Bailey, 1977)

POSSIBLE PERSONAL AND SOCIAL ASPECTS OF STRESS

Kogan and colleagues (1971) in their study 'Working Relationships within the British Hospital Service' produced an analysis concerning the working relationships of the nursing and medical staff. The relationship between doctors and nurses is described as a 'prescribing/treatment' relationship. It is contrasted with the superior/subordinate relationships that are part of other work situations in which the superior has the responsibility and accountability for the whole of the subordinate's work activity. In the prescribing/treatment relationship the doctor is seen as accountable only for ensuring that specific treatment is performed, not for the whole of the other's work activity.

This concept is of interest particularly when looking at what happens in operating theatres. It would appear to suggest that the nurses might well be considered by the prescribing staff much as a piece of theatre equipment to be used for a specific purpose, in this case the performance of an operation. Such a depersonalising attitude, should it exist, can only be based on lack of understanding of the purpose and function of the whole hospital organisation and could well have a damaging effect on work performance and morale and increase stress within the operating theatre. Role perception, both of self and of others, is necessary to the well-being of any organisation (Rowbottom, 1973; Revans, 1972; Robson, 1986) and, unless all role activities are recognised as purposes for which the organisation exists, the organisation will be defective (Kogan et al, 1971). The concept also offers an understanding of a possible area of stress-producing conflict in operating theatres, for should there be a suggestion in the real work situation of lack of mutual awareness of each other's function within the organisation, confusion and conflict will arise. Satisfactory fulfilment of work requirements depends upon satisfactory self-fulfilment of the individual committed to the production of those work requirements, which in turn depends on the understanding and knowledge of a particular environment (Revans, 1972; Drucker, 1967; Maslow, 1943). This is the case when the work required is safe, efficient and kind patient care, as with any other work requirement. The statement of aims and objectives of an organisation, whether general or specific, short- or long-term, small or large scale, helps to promote both knowledge and understanding and in so doing improves morale and lessens stress (Pollitt, 1977). Health-care aims and objectives can cover anything from the philosophical statements concerning the nursing practices of a particular hospital (Hoeller, 1974) to the relatively short-term objectives of training needs (Nolan, 1975; Fish, 1974) or, as is the case with the quoted statement at the start of this chapter, the 'raison d'être' of a specific group within an organisation. The achievement of aims and objectives requires the knowledge, under-standing, hard work and willingness to partake of all those in-volved. It has to be borne in mind that complaints about the physical aspects of an environment may be disguised complaints against organisational aspects, just as inadequate structural environments can house teams with high morale (Lunn, 1975; Revans, 1972).

POSSIBLE ENVIRONMENTAL ASPECTS OF STRESS

The physical environment of the operating theatre has undergone over the years continuous modification and development and, although the hospitals in Britain are using operating theatres that are at varying points on the modification and development scale, the indications are, not surprisingly, that the ideal environment is continually being sought within the available budgets (Phillips, 1980; Hughes, 1981). The operating theatre can be an up-to-the-minute, sealed, modular unit (Hughes, 1981) or the result of continuing adaption of existing accommodation to the technologies and techniques of modern day surgery.

One of the controversial casualties of up-dating was the loss of windows from operating theatre design as internal lighting systems improved. Lunn (1975) sees the disappearance of windows from operating theatres as a benefit. Their presense affected the internal temperature for they were a source of radiant heat in hot weather and caused problems of heat loss when it was cold. Stress problems associated with low morale have now been reported that are seen as being related to the lack of windows (Phillips, 1980). Greaves (1974) stated that, although work commencement in a new and windowless theatre had been regarded as a potential problem, the staff reaction within the work environment had been favourable. This ambivalence would appear to reinforce the psychosocial determinants of a team or work group described by several authorities (Nichols et al, 1981; Gatley, 1981; Pollitt, 1977) and it would also appear to emphasise how interrelated are the environ-mental, personal and social aspects of stress.

Temperature is an environmental factor in the work situation that is of great importance. The optimum temperature and relative humidity are found to vary little in discussions in the literature (Lamont, 1977). The safety of the patient, the comfort of 'scrubbed' personnel (Lamont, 1977), the control of static electricity (Brigden, 1974) and the inhibition of possible bacterial growth (Lunn, 1975) are all factors that contribute to the acceptability of a temperature between 21°C (68°F) and 22°C (72°F), with a humidity of between 50% and 60%. The age and condition of the patient should also influence the temperature required, the very young and the very old often requiring a warmer environment.

Stephens and Boaler's work (1977) brought to the notice of those interested in the problems of operating theatres that their study area had theatre units not only without recovery rooms but also without postoperative recovery nurses. Recovery and reception areas provide safety for patients in that their very specific needs are catered for. The presence of such areas lessens stress for both medical and nursing staff because the requirements for patient care, both pre- and postoperatively, are to hand. It has not always been realised that the position of these areas within the theatre department is of significance. Greaves (1974) and Phillips (1980) both point out that the placing of these areas has implications for the quality of the patient's care at a time when he is at his most vulnerable. The reception area should not be part of the general access to the operating theatre and it should be well away from office and rest room noise, as well as being nowhere near the sights and sounds of a recovery area.

Theatre sterile supply units are now part of the basic design of an operating department, either within it or situated in such a manner that there is a direct communication, for example, a supply lift between floors. Phillips (1980) discusses the problems of large multi-suite operating theatres, not only in terms of actual physical distance but also with respect to the psychosocial distances that can occur between staff in the department as a whole, including the theatre sterile supply unit, and the possible resultant management difficulties.

The ventilation of operating theatres and the use of exhaust systems to rid the environment of the exhaled anaesthetic gases (Charnley, 1970; Howorth, 1981) provide vast subject areas. A larger study could usefully include an analysis of the air of operating theatres in relation to staff experience of stress.

An understanding of the work environment is a necessary element in the control of stress. Most of the literature reviewed here has been written by staff working within the operating department indicating, it is suggested, that there is an awareness among interested nurses of what contributes to the success or failure of their organisation, its satisfaction and its stresses. The two broad areas indicated in this review are considered in the research proper as possible sources of conflict; one area was described as being subjective and seen to equate with possible personal and social aspects of the work situation, and the other area was described as objective and seen to equate with certain design and management aspects of the work situation.

5 | The operating list

The operating list may be regarded as a mutually accepted agreed way of planning to achieve the aim of safe patient care. It is the means whereby the organisation of the operating theatre and the relevant wards (remembering that one operating theatre can receive patients from several wards, and one ward supply patients to several operating theatres) is planned for routine operating sessions. The operating list is the visible sign of co-operation and agreement between those who will be using it as a basis for their plan of work. Thus it is the focus of organisation for nursing and medical staff, X-ray, pathology and haematology departments, as well as for the internal transport and portering systems within the hospital. Within the hospital organisation there is an assumption that the order of the operating list is to be relied upon. Indeed, the list would be valueless as an instrument of organisation if this were not the case. But the operating list is vulnerable to change. There are many reasons why this is so, all reflections of the inherent instability of the hospital environment (Pembrey, 1980). It is accepted that some changes are unavoidable (Medical Defence Union and Royal College of Nursing, 1978; Department of Health and Social Security, 1970), such as deterioration in a patient's condition, making cancellation necessary. Whatever the reason, nurses remain very aware of the added risk to patients when changes to the order of the operating list occur (Campbell, 1979; Dixon, 1978; Brett, 1976; Cox, 1974; Hassell, 1971).

One reason for the frequently experienced organisational problems which are not always related to clinical emergencies (Revans, 1972) is that, in spite of its deceptively simple tactical format, the operating list conceals the differing priorities and purposes of the two main groups of staff who deal directly with the patients on that operating list at the point of delivery of care. These are the medical and nursing staff who subdivide into four groups:

1.   the surgeons;
2.   the anaesthetists;
3.   the theatre nursing staff;
4.   the ward nursing staff.

These groups approach the patient with the same aim but with different priorities. They all work within the prescriber/treatment working relationship (Kogan et al, 1971) which becomes extremely complex in the operating theatre as the role positions constantly change between the staff groups, depending on the exigencies of the moment. If the specific and particular clinical skills and expertise of the four main groups are set on one side and consideration given to some of the organisational aspects of the immediate work environment, a diagrammatic representation can be constructed that gives some indication of the complexity of pressures experienced by staff at the point of delivery of patient care. Few, if any, of these 'pressures' will be the same. For instance, all groups have teaching responsibilities but they are all different teaching responsibilities, so there is the possibility of an increase in the stress as one group resists the pressure of the other. The availability of suitable nursing staff may clash with the need to get a waiting list 'down', and so on. Figure 3 represents the organisational pressures present while attending to one patient at one point in time on one operating list.

The reality of the situation is of course more complex than this, for the same organisational pressures may be assumed to have existed for the patient preceding, as well as the one following, the hypothetical patient of the diagram who is undergoing surgery in a single theatre. In twin theatres the pressures are multiplied and in multi-theatre suites, which in the UK may contain up to 21 theatres, pressures will increase accordingly, as does the possibility of hazard to the patient (Phillips, 1980).

The pressure/priority lists in the diagram (Figure 3) are not exhaustive, nor are they intended to be. The intention is only that they should indicate the complexities of organisation in the environment surrounding the working through of an operating list and the possibilities present for conflict and stress in the personnel involved (Elliott, 1966).

Lazarus (1964) describes 'states of stress' as generally attending

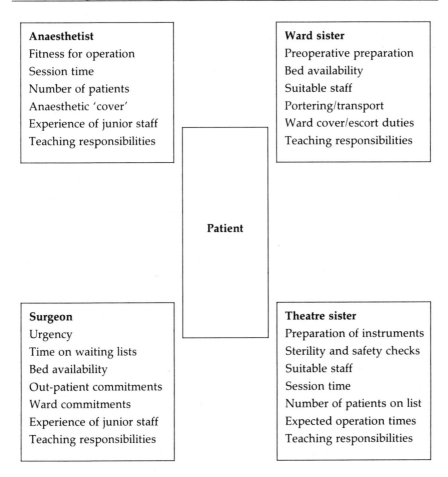

Figure 3 An indication of some organisational pressures on surgeons, anaesthetists, theatre nurses and ward nurses at the point of surgical intervention

the conflict occurring when powerful motives are thwarted. The aim of safe patient surgery is a powerful motivating force in all the staff concerned. As Revans (1972) says, it is in the 'manner of doing' that stress will occur, for priorities do differ and conflict of interest will arise. The behavioural aspects of this are accepted as part of the 'norm' of the high stress area of an operating theatre. The staff working in such an area are those who are able to work intelligently and coherently, carrying out the work activities of their particular group in these particular circumstances. But there remain areas of stress in their work environment that are seen by nurses as avoidable. Such areas may be problems of structure and design, or be caused by the interpersonal relationships and role relationships of those involved. Other difficulties arise when there is apparent, in some staff, a lack of awareness of the absolute need for the efficient use of the scarce manpower and time resources within operating theatres (Brett, 1978).

Manpower and time are scarce and expensive resources in the National Health Service and the operating list is a system that utilises both in order to provide the required service to the patient. The introduction of the 37½-hour working week for nurses would appear to have exacerbated a situation in which manpower had already been recognised as limited (Department of Heath and Social Security, 1974). The importance of cost-effective use of limited resources is recognised by many members of the nursing and medical professions (Aries, 1981; Carr, 1978; Stephens and Boaler, 1977; Hunter, 1972). Methods are evolving of calculating workload information in order to assist with the organisation of the manpower needs of operating theatres (Freeman, 1976) and wards (Rhys-Hearn, 1972; Barr, 1967). The theatre nursing staff in charge of the running of an operating list are the managers of the scarce manpower and time resources (Campbell, 1979; Dixon, 1978; Cranfield, 1972) and it is the successful co-ordination of these that enables surgery to take place safely and efficiently.

Success or lack of success in controlling the list within its session is seen as an important indication of managerial ability in operating theatres (Hulme, 1973). Indeed, reference to both professional and personal satisfaction in relation to the working of the list is to be found in the literature (Ross, 1977; Bosanquet, 1974). The more frequently occurring references, however, are to stress experiences (Phillips, 1980; Revans, 1972; Hassell, 1971). Assuming that those who continue to work in operating theatres are those to whom the inevitable stress of the presenting situation is taken as a challenge, adding interest and zest to life (Coleman, 1978; Pollitt, 1977; Selye, 1965, 1978), it is suggested that the stresses mentioned in the literature and described as having a bad effect on morale are those perceived as avoidable by staff, and which occur over and above the accepted level of stress. It would appear possible that one answer to the presence of avoidable stress in the operating theatre might be found in the use to which the scarce resources of manpower and time are put, and their management within the complex role-relationships of the work situation.

The function of managing contains mixtures of balance of responsibility, authority and accountability (both up and down within the organisation) as well as control, leadership and the realisation of the motivational and developmental requirements of the individual, and communication needs (Handy, 1985; Maslow, 1943, 1970; Drucker, 1967; Likert, 1961; McGregor, 1957). Management theory and philosophy are wide and continually developing areas; the scope of the present study allows for a mere indication of their application in considering some of the presenting problems connected with stress and nursing staff in operating theatres.

Coghill (1972) describes a manager as someone who may work at any level within an organisation and is able to spot problems and find solutions, adding the rider that solutions can only be implemented if the organisation itself is properly trained. For an organisation to work properly both the 'managers' and the 'managed' must understand the aims and objectives of the organisation and their function within it (Handy, 1985; Robson, 1986). Coghill further points out that development within the health service is an index of its ability to assimilate new ideas and technologies as well as an indication of its ability to modify the working environment to improve patient care. One aspect of this is discussed in the work of Davies (1972) in which she examines the reason for the failure of the National Health Service Management Course as a means of assimilating management philosophies and theories. Failure to understand the nature of the changing environment (Archer et al, 1984), the roles and role-perception of self and others or the personal and professional requirements within a system leads to confusion and conflict and to deep anxieties and mistrust concerning the unstable areas, the state described as 'parataxis' by Revans (1971). The functional aspects of the operating list present one such unstable area (Hunter, 1972; Hindle, 1970).

Although it is the theatre nurse in charge who is described as managing the operating list during its 'running through' within the allowed time it is the surgeon, for obvious reasons, who controls the number of patients who are to be operated on within a particular session. This is the liaison area mentioned by both the Briggs and Lewin Reports that is of significance in maintaining good relationships within the operating theatre. The average length of an operation is a factor of considerable relevance to staffing needs in the operating theatre, as it is on the wards (Revans, 1972). Surgeons are noted for their optimistic estimations of operation times (Hindle, 1970). Good communication with both the theatre and the ward staff is essential if problems are to be avoided. The pressure against cancelling a patient's operation is immense, for there is complete awareness of all the requirements and preparation necessary for a routine admission, starting with arrangements concerning work and home commitments and finishing with the giving of the pre-medication. When goodwill exists and there are established working relationships any system will work, all groups adjusting to the give and take of a particular situation. However, in the changing hospitals of today and the larger complexes of staff concentrations and facilities, staff mobility is high and the established working relationship may be rare.

Effective communication is a key-point in considering resource use and avoidable stress in operating theatres. Brett in 1978, eight years after the Lewin recommendations in favour of the establishment of multidisciplinary theatre-user committees, asked how many such committees there were in existence at that point which were viable and had proper representation of all the grades of staff who worked in the operating theatres. She further asked if any attempt at all had been made to rationalise the operating theatre services and to improve the conditions of service, thereby reducing stress for patients and staff alike. Rait in 1976, while in full agreement that the theatre-user committees were not working as had been envisaged, felt that Lewin's main achievement had been to cause a division between doctors and nurses working in operating theatres, a division certainly demonstrated in Dixon's (1978) statement that, while some doctors agreed that staff working in the theatre were more vulnerable to legal action than in other areas, the majority of doctors saw no reason to give special consideration to their needs. When attitudes such as this are acknowledged to exist within a powerful professional body it can come as no surprise to realise that nursing staff anxiety may deepen to mistrust should organisational changes or difficulties arise and stress levels become intolerable.

In this chapter some functional aspects of the operating list have been discussed. The working relationships and differing priorities of those at the point of delivery of care have been indicated. This part of the study literature review would appear to suggest that opportunities for stress over and above acceptable levels to staff may be related to the organisation of the operating list.

6 | The patient, the nurse and stress

It is hardly surprising to discover that the available literature supports the view that the prospect of surgery is stressful for the patient (Wilson-Barnett, 1979; Boore, 1978; Janis, 1958). Not only is surgery frightening in itself, bringing the individual into contact with feared experiences of pain and helplessness, but also it has an impact on the patient's view of himself and his body (Gruendemann, 1975). In recent years the growing awareness within the nursing profession of the necessity for individual patient care (Heath and Law, 1981; Roper et al, 1980; McFarlane, 1978) has resulted in studies examining what is done to patients in the name of nursing care, and why.

The continuity of care for the patient is the objective of nursing staff in operating theatres as elsewhere in hospitals (Campbell, 1979; Brett, 1976; Dixon, 1976). Within the relative isolation of the operating theatre the elements of nursing (Roper et al, 1980) are brought into sharper focus as the patient consents to relinquish the control of his activities of living (Henderson, 1966) to the care of those supporting him at this most vulnerable time.

Studies undertaken by nurses into the nursing care that patients receive have added to the research-based body of knowledge that is replacing traditionally-based care concepts (McFarlane, 1978). Anxiety and its psychological and physiological results can be considerably lessened by preoperative information (Boore, 1978; Murphy et al, 1977; Hayward, 1975) and it has been proved that giving of information has a significant effect on postoperative pain and recovery rates in patients, as well as on their postoperative infection rate. Information relies upon communication to make it come alive and work. Should communication systems not be able to handle the information available, either in the broad and general parameters of continuing education and self-development, or in the

33

more specific and local parameters of person-to-person communication, the information, however appropriate, will become lifeless or valueless. Hunter (1972) analyses the situation in which gaps in the nurse's information (in this particular instance the reason for change in the planned organisation of the day) adversely influence the length of the patient's stay in hospital. Communication failure may result in incorrect premedication times as well as excessive preoperative starvation, problems also associated with inaccurate information and general lack of awareness of information and its importance in the function of the organisation (Hunter, 1972).

The essential emotional and physical preparedness of the patient for surgery, his well-being and safety, are to be found in the individual approach to his care. The logical approach to preoperative preparation, comfort and support and preoperative medications can only be on an individual basis (Lewin, 1978; Shepherd, 1976; Norris and Campbell, 1975; Hamilton-Smith, 1972; Baxter, 1971; Cox, 1974). There would appear to be three main areas of difficulty concerning the care of the patient on the day of operation, causes of anxiety to both the patient and the nurse, namely:

1. patient anxiety at delay and change;
2. incorrect premedication timings;
3. excessive preoperative starvation.

PATIENT ANXIETY AT DELAY AND CHANGE

Improved resource use and service of care to the patient are seen as essential in the reduction of stress for patients and staff (Brett, 1978). Delays and alterations to the operating list do not constitute improvement of service to the patient or good use of resources and can create both a nerve-racking and a dangerous experience for the individual patient concerned (Baxter, 1971; Phillips, 1980). Patients like to know when they will have their operation, how long it is likely to take and when they are likely to be back in bed on the ward. Anxieties at delays and changes can be quite severe, and a positive relationship between preoperative anxiety and the postoperative state has been demonstrated (Hayward, 1975; Janis, 1958). It is stressful for nursing staff who are attempting to provide the correct preoperative environment for the patient of informed support and quiet to discover not only that the organisation of the events in the patient's day is beyond their control, but also that the information they may have to work with is either inadequate or non-existent (Hunter, 1972). Information is power and status, and the withholding of it indicates the lack of status that both nurses and their patients are accorded in the organisation.

It has been said that nurses in the operating theatre have not been very good at explaining to their nursing colleagues in other areas of the hospital what it is that they actually do that is important to continuing patient care (O'Connor, 1971). Nurses, whether in the theatre or elsewhere, have not always been skilled at this type of communication. One aspect of what theatre nurses 'do' may be found in their awareness of the need to minimise patient anxiety in the preoperative period by attempting to ensure that the scheduling of the operating list is as planned. This might provide one reason as to why the nursing staff in the operating theatre state that they experience intense anxiety at changes to the operating list, particularly the order in which the patients are scheduled to arrive (Phillips, 1980). Nolan in 1975 indicated that evaluation of care in the operating rooms of North America has a financial aspect. She stated that an evaluation of what is done by nurses for the patient in the operating room is required in order that the consumer, that is the patient, can be assured that he is getting the 'nursing he needs, wants and is paying for'. Unnecessary anxieties will be recognised as a fall in nursing quality and may well be echoed in a similar financial fall.

INCORRECT PREMEDICATION TIMING

Premedication may be given to a patient for the following reasons (Norris and Campbell, 1975):

1. to relieve anxiety, which may also include pain relief;
2. to abolish or reduce undesirable parasympathetic activity;
3. to reduce postoperative vomiting.

It is recognised that the relief of anxiety, or sedation, nowadays is the most important function of premedication. In those patients in whom pain is present preoperatively, anxiety may well be relieved by the alleviation of pain but in routine, elective surgery, psychic sedation or anxiety relief is the main objective (Norris and

Campbell, 1975). The timing of the premedication is of the utmost importance. The non-irritant solutions of the opiates and atropine may be given by subcutaneous injection 1–1½ hours pre-operatively, the somewhat more irritant substances by intra-muscular injection 30–40 minutes preoperatively. It is useless and possibly dangerous to give a premedication at a time before the induction of the anaesthetic when it cannot be absorbed (Norris and Campbell, 1975). The giving of the premedication at the appropriate time is part of the preoperative care provided by the nursing staff on the ward. It is something that requires planning and good liaison between the ward and theatre staffs if such an individual measure is to be used well. The use of oral premedication precludes anxieties concerning exact premedication timings (Norris and Campbell, 1975). These are effective for up to four hours so, for a routine list, not only is the timing not such a critical factor for the individual, but also any changes in scheduling can be absorbed without stress because most of the patients will have received their oral pre-medication before the operating list commences.

EXCESSIVE PREOPERATIVE STARVATION

The study by Hamilton-Smith (1972) indicated that routine preoper-ative fasting or starvation times varied considerably and that there was little evidence other than tradition on which these varying practices were based. A four-hour term during which fluids, food and sweets are withheld is a general rule (Norris and Campbell, 1975) but up to twelve-hour periods of planned starvation have been recorded (Hamilton-Smith, 1972). This variation alone is fraught with physiological difficulties for the patient, but the problem becomes one of increasing danger should preoperative starvation be carried out on successive days due to unavoidable cancellations (Hunter, 1972).

There are also circumstances which have a slowing effect on gastric emptying, circumstances which may well have influenced some of the longer planned starvation times mentioned. For instance, should a limb be broken soon after a meal has been eaten the stomach has been known to take up to 10 hours to empty. Preg-nancy has a slowing effect on the rate of emptying, as does anxiety. A further aspect of the problem of preoperative starvation is that a liver which is short of glycogen is more susceptible to infection and the effect of hepatotoxic substances formed by some anaesthetic drugs. Illness, trauma and starvation increase demands on the nutritional stores of the body (Hamilton-Smith, 1972) and difficulties may also be encountered with fluid and electrolyte balance (Campbell, 1979; Hamilton-Smith, 1972).

The literature discussed in this chapter has been that in which the essential requirements for individual patient care have been considered, and the three areas of preoperative care that can only ever be individual have been discussed, namely:

1.   patient anxiety at delay and change;
2.   incorrect premedication timing;
3.   excessive preoperative starvation.

These literature review chapters are intended to indicate that the stresses and strains of everyday life in Western society are at a high level even before an individual commences in one of the many stressful occupations. Nursing, although not heading the list of stressful occupations, is recognised as being one such and it is acknowledged that there are particular areas within nursing that are seen as being more stress-producing than others. Some elements influencing the work in operating theatres have been discussed and these include aspects of the working relationships, the design and the organisation. The preoperative care of the patient, the prerogative of the ward staff but vulnerable to change as a direct result of the activity within the operating theatre, has been considered as part of the nurse–patient caring relationship. There would appear to be many different reasons why stress may be the experience of the nurse who has the care of the patient on his day of operation.

Part II: The research

7 Aims and objectives

HYPOTHESES

The two hypotheses being explored in this study were:

1. that the qualified nurse who has the care of the patient on his day of operation in the theatre or in the ward experiences additional stress should a change or changes occur in the expected organisation of the day;
2. that there is a relationship between the experience of the nurses in theatre and the experience of the nursing staff in the ward.

UNDERLYING ASSUMPTIONS

The main assumptions underlying these hypotheses included:

1. that stress has a detrimental effect on staff morale;
2. that a relationship has been shown to exist between poor staff morale and longer patient recovery rates (Revans, 1964);
3. that staff working in areas regarded as stressful are those who are able to cope with the 'normal' stresses of the day;
4. that stress perceived by staff as stress experience is over and above the expected 'normal' stress levels of the working day;
5. that stress relating to the patient will be more intense than other stresses;
6. that stress experience ranges from the merely irritating to the catastrophic.

41

AIMS AND OBJECTIVES

The aims and objectives formulated to assist in the validation or rejection of the hypotheses reflect both staff experience of stress and staff experience of satisfaction. By these means it was hoped to achieve a more balanced view of the whole experience of the day, for satisfaction is as much a part of the nursing day as is stress (Nichols et al, 1981; The Committee on Nursing, 1972). The study aims and objectives as well as the reasoning underlying their choice are listed below.

1. *To establish the existence of elements contributing to nursing staff stress in operating theatres*
Without this basic information the study would be meaningless. There has always been much general awareness among nurses, an awareness reflected in the relevant literature reviewed in the earlier chapters, that various factors do contribute to stress experienced by operating theatre nurses. The need in this study was to establish the existence of possible stress-producing elements in the operating theatres.

2. *To establish perception of stress experience in theatre nursing staff*
Experience of stress is individual: that which might cause anxiety in one person may pass unnoticed by another. One of the controls on the amount of information to be collected in this study was that the experience of one person only, the qualified nurse in charge of the work of the routine list, would be collected. This meant of course that only one viewpoint would be noted for each session. The study maximum would be 40 people from within the study population of four different health authorities. Intensity of the stress experience would also be noted.

3. *To establish perception of satisfaction experience in theatre nursing staff*
Stress and satisfaction are both part of the experience of the nurse's working day. Experience is individual and, as with stress, awareness of experience may well differ in perception and intensity. The 'satisfaction' information was to be collected directly from each individual nurse identified as a sample number and recorded similarly to the 'stress' information.

4. *To establish perception of stress experience in ward nursing staff*

As with stress in theatre nursing staff it was first of all necessary to establish the existence of stress perception in ward staff in order to be able to consider the two main hypotheses of this study.

5. *To establish perception of satisfaction experience in ward nursing staff*

Again, the satisfaction information is a basic requirement in this study of stress in operating theatres and wards during routine operating lists. Information about the positive as well as the negative aspects of the day is felt to be required in order that a balanced overview of the perception of the working environment may be established.

6. *To establish a possible relationship between the experience of the theatre and the wards*

RESEARCH SUBJECTS

The target population was identified as all those qualified nursing staff who had the care of the patient on his day of operation within the selected hospitals. The sample population available for this study was the one qualified nurse, state registered or state enrolled, who was the nurse in overall charge of the patient in the operating theatre, and the one qualified nurse in charge on the ward during a particular routine operating list in each of the theatres and wards of the study hospitals. Thus, the nurses who took part in this study shared the following characteristics:

- all were qualified nurses;
- all cared for the patient either in the theatre or on the ward;
- each one was the nurse who had the overall responsibility and authority for the patient's care in either the theatre or the ward;
- all were caring for patients during the working-through of routine operating lists.

The sample from which the accessible sample population was taken was provided by the relevant nursing staff of five different area health authorities. This, it was hoped, would provide a sample size that would be considered realistic. The choice of area health authorities was one of convenience: I had either trained or worked as a qualified member of staff in each one of them. A further, larger study of the same field of work would of course use random selection techniques.

The response rate of the accessible population for the sample was 100% as the research was planned and executed in order to achieve that response. Individuals, theatres and hospitals were all offered the chance to withdraw if they so wished but none did. Contingency plans contained a reserve hospital should there be withdrawals but this was not required. The observations, interviews and recording were carried out by one person, myself.

8 The research design and method

THE RESEARCH DESIGN

The purpose of research design is to guide both the collection and the analysis of data in such a way that the results yielded are interpretable and generisable to the larger target population (Polit and Hungler, 1978). The strongest of the designs for this purpose are experimental (Polit and Hungler, 1978). Control and experimental groups are capable of manipulation in planned 'before' and 'after' situations, manoeuvres that are not always feasible in nursing for a variety of reasons ranging from the ethical to the practical. The design of the present research is non-experimental. It is a descriptive and exploratory piece of research (Clark and Hockey, 1979; Diers, 1979) and is seen as a pilot study providing an information base for further research. The control of the research in this study was exerted through the selection of a suitable sample to provide the subject material for the study and by the appropriateness of the research tool developed for the information collection.

The most significant constraints on the design of this research were the time available, the associated financial implications and the fact that there was only one person to undertake the research, all quite common constraints, particularly for nurses. The research had to be planned several months in advance of commencement in order that letters of introduction and explanation could be received and answered by the hospitals selected (see appendix I for a copy of the letter). As staff stress only was being explored patient involvement would be indirect and minimal. The permission to allow this study to be conducted was requested from and granted by the

45

nursing and medical consultant staff in all the involved hospitals. Ethical committee decisions, although always a possibility, were not required in this study (Downie and Calman, 1987).

The sample of hospitals chosen for this study may be described as a sample of convenience. A full-size research project in this field would use randomisation to choose the sample areas as a means of control (Polit and Hungler, 1978). In order to exert some control on the situation to be studied and also to provide a wide view of current practice in the relevant area, hospitals within five different area health authorities were contacted, and all were pleased to be able to co-operate in the research. The criterion for choice was the fact that I had at some point worked in each hospital, either as a learner or as a trained member of staff. This was found to produce a useful introduction not only to the nursing staff in general but also to the subject groups in particular, and it was of immense personal interest to me to see the developments, or lack of them, that had occurred in the intervening years.

Once the decision had been taken concerning the number of hospitals in the study and their letters of acceptance had been received, some idea of the study size could be gained. Routine operating sessions were to provide the work environment; emergency surgery carries with it different pressures. There was suffcient time to allow for one five-day working week pre-pilot study and four five-day working weeks for the study itself. A morning or afternoon session would be categorised as one routine session. An all-day session, that is using both morning and afternoon session time, would also be classed as one routine session. This would allow a maximum of 40 routine sessions to be observed during the four-week study planned. Consultation with the staff of the University of Manchester Computation Department indicated that the data yielded from a study of this size would be suitable for statistical analysis by computer. A basic time schedule was devised.

- *Week 1* Pre-pilot study at first hospital in order to develop and modify research tool.
- *Weeks 2-5* Data collection at hospitals in study. First data to computer for card punching.
- *Week 6* Kept in reserve with fall-back arrangements with first hospital should an unexpected cancellation occur.
- *Weeks 7-10* Completion of card punching. Preliminary computer statistical analysis of data.

- *Weeks 11-16* Interpretation of statistical analysis of data. Writing-up of research.

The arrangement for week 6 was felt to be essential in view of the time constraints and the related size of the research project. In fact, at the last hospital there were administrative difficulties that nearly caused these fall-back arrangements to be required. The five weeks allowed for interpretation of the data and writing up proved, not surprisingly, to be totally unrealistic. Far, far more time was required.

THE RESEARCH METHOD

A research method is the technique used to collect and order data (Treece and Treece, 1977). Research methods used for the study of nurses and their work, limited because of the nature of nursing (Sweeney and Olivieri, 1981), generally include interview schedules, questionnaires, ranking systems and direct observation (Polit and Hungler, 1978). Two of the above methods are used in this study – the observational method and the interview schedule.

Observational method

Observational methods are techniques for acquiring information for research purposes through the direct observation and interpretation of phenomena in the environment. Polit and Hungler (1978) demonstrate six classes of phenomena that are amenable to observational study:

1. verbal communication behaviours;
2. non-verbal communication behaviours;
3. actions and activities;
4. skill attainment and performance;
5. characteristics, attributes or conditions of individuals;
6. environmental characteristics.

Observation of environmental characteristics was felt to be an appropriate data-collecting method for this present descriptive and exploratory piece of research concerning some aspects of stress in nursing staff on operating days.

Observational methodology has both advantages and disadvantages, strengths and weaknesses, and any research plan should be prepared to consider both the negative and the positive aspects of the methodology chosen. As Treece and Treece (1977) point out, research findings are always at the mercy of the methods and techniques used to obtain them. The choice of an appropriate methodology in relation to the type of research planned is of significance when considering the strength of the internal validity of the research findings.

The central appeal of observational methodology is that it is possible to capture directly a record of the events of the moment in depth and variety, and also to have sufficient flexibility to be able to allow for either an experimental or a non-experimental approach. Polit and Hungler (1978) state that, within the area of nursing research, 'observational methods have broad applicability for clinical enquiries, as well as for educational and administrative studies'.

The disadvantages of observational methodology are those to be found in an analysis of the observer/observed relationship in any observation. These include ethical problems, the possible reaction of the observed when the observer is present and lack of consent of those involved. There is also a continuous threat to the validity of the research findings because of the possibility of significant observer-identification producing problems of distortion and bias affecting data interpretation.

Bearing in mind that there were disadvantages as well as advantages in the choice, the decision to use the observational method of collecting and recording data was made. A further decision concerning what type of observer/observed relationship would be most appropriate to the requirements of the research had to be made. There are four possibilities here. The observer/observed relationship may be:

1.   concealment/no intervention;
2.   no concealment/no intervention;
3.   no concealment/intervention;
4.   concealment/intervention.

A matrix created by the intersection of an intervention/no intervention continuum and a concealment/no concealment continuum indicates some of the possible difficulties that might be encountered using an observer/observed observational methodology. As is demonstrated in figure 4 concealment of the observer is a source of ethical problems and presence of the observer is a

Intervention

Ethical problems (lack of consent, of privacy)	Reaction to observer Entry permission problems
Different behaviour due to intervention	Different behaviour due to intervention
Possible superficiality	Observer bias due to identification

Concealment	**No concealment**
Ethical problems (lack of consent, of privacy)	Reaction to observer Entry permission problems
Low incidence of behaviour of interest in natural setting	Low incidence of behaviour of interest in natural setting
Reduced ability to infer causal relationships	Reduced ability to infer causal relationships
Possible superficiality	Observer bias due to identification

No intervention

Figure 4   Possible problems in observer/observed relationship (after Polit and Hungler, 1978)

source of possible observer-reaction or observer-identification.

The type of observer/observed relationship chosen for this present study was that of 'no concealment/ no intervention', a position having much in common with the participant observation used in anthropology and sociology (Polit and Hungler, 1978). The observer would be present within the situation and the subject group would know the reason for the presence of the observer. Exchange of information and discussion would take place but the observer, although part of the subject group's social activities, such as conversation and meals, would be outside the professional activities, the work of the operating day.

Interview schedule

Polit and Hungler (1978) describe the personal interview as being the most powerful method of securing information because of the depth and quality of information that is yielded. The information about individual perception of stress and satisfaction was to be collected from the staff using a simple interview schedule. The interview in this study was conceived as being as informal as possible to encourage discussion. It was hoped that, by opening with a leading remark concerning the experience of the day and following with simple questions about the 'good' and 'difficult' aspects of the day, an indication of staff experience of stress and satisfaction would be acquired. A rating scale (Polit and Hungler, 1978) was included in order that an indication of staff perception of the intensity of the experience might be recorded. This weighting should, it was felt, create a more realistic overview of the stresses and satisfactions of the day by balancing minor irritations against more major experiences rather than a mere counting of occurrences.

9 The construction of the research tool and the pre-pilot study

The creation of a suitable research tool or instrument is an essential step in any research and as such requires a basic understanding of the aims and objectives of the planned area of study (Polit and Hungler, 1978). The instrument created should be as simple as possible, present as unbiased a stimulus to the user or users as possible, and also present as professional appearance as possible (Sweeney and Olivieri, 1981). Consultation and testing should contribute to its modification during development (Sweeney and Olivieri, 1981; Polit and Hungler, 1978) and the research tool should be capable not only of collecting the relevant information but also of collecting it in a manner that renders it suitable for any subsequent analysis.

The aims and objectives of this study (see chapter 7) required a collection instrument on which to record, during the working-through of a routine operation list, the following information:

- certain environmental, administrative and structural design elements in the operating theatre;
- stress perception and intensity in operating theatre nurses;
- satisfaction perception and intensity in operating theatre nurses;
- stress perception and intensity in ward staff;
- satisfaction perception and intensity in ward staff.

The two types of information just described require that the information collecting tool be in two parts: one part designed to record the information which would be observed, and the second part designed to record the information collected during the informal interviews. The construction of a simple collection method for the objective factual information proved to be straightforward, the only constraints being that:

- the information should be relevant to the study;
- the information should be that which could be collected by one person during a routine operating list.

To this end a check-list of possible elements for consideration within the theatre environment was made, which had to be tested and modified as necessary during the planned pre-pilot study working week of Monday to Friday (see appendix II for check-list). The supporting reasons for the inclusion of any item of information on this preliminary list were that:

- the item had been mentioned in the literature reviewed for this study as contributing to stress;
- the item was regarded in general by theatre nursing staff as having a significant influence upon the experience of the day.

During the testing of the efficiency of the preliminary check-list as a possible research instrument considerable modification and development occurred, far more than had been foreseen. The preliminary check-list for the collection of the factual environmental information became a formal three-page document in which the original list had been expanded and a system for organising the information for computer analysis was added (see appendix III). Table 1 lists those items included for consideration, and which are described as the objective variables in this study.

The items finally chosen do not represent an exhaustive list by any means. During the testing and modification of the research instrument it was realised that to keep this exploratory study to a reasonable size there would have to be certain limits set to the number of items for inclusion as study variables. For instance, classification of operations would be major, intermediate or minor, choices relying on the local policy of the theatre and hospital. (Some hospital policies do not recognise the category of 'minor'.) Speciality would not be noted. Patients would only be considered numerically; neither age nor sex would be included. There would be no distinction made between in-patient and day-case categories of patient. This approach was intended to limit the amount of information

Table 1 List of environmental and organisational elements in this study described as the objective variables

Time allowed	Presence/absence of receptionist or reception area
Time taken	Theatre temperature
Delayed start	Theatre humidity
Number of operations	Perception of theatre temperature
Number and types of operation	Presence/absence of window(s)
Control of premedication time	Type of theatre (single, twin, multi-suite)
Control of operation time	
Alterations to list	Staff shared between theatres
Additions to list	Standard swab, needle and instrument counting/recording procedures
Cancellations to list	
Order of list changed	
Inaccuracies in list	
Uncommunicated changes to list	Number of qualified staff
Number of alterations to list	Number of theatre-experienced qualified staff
Morning list delivered the previous afternoon	
	Seniority of nurse in charge
Afternoon list delivered the previous afternoon	Number of learner nurses
	Learners as part of work force
List typed	Number of nursing auxiliaries
Patient crisis	'On-call' staff
Presence/absence of theatre sterile supply unit	Staff expected to stay late
	Meal breaks
Presence/absence of recovery room	Observed signs of stress (verbal and non-verbal)

to be handled as well as allowing a fairly wide range of possible environmental influences to be considered. Should analysis indicate that a particular area would repay further study, the information for that study could be expanded at a later date to allow for a more thorough investigation. It was realised, though, that limiting the information available for analysis might possibly conceal relevant elements.

The second type of information required for this study was that to be collected during the informal interviews planned to take place at the conclusion of each routine operating session. There would be only one nurse interviewed in the theatre and one in the ward, and that would be the qualified nurse in charge of the particular session. The information collected from these interviews would form the subjective variables. The concept forming the constructional basis of the informal interview is one discussed by J C Flanagan in his study 'The critical incident technique' (1954). In his study this technique is described as a set of procedures for collecting direct observations of human behaviour in such a way as 'to facilitate their potential usefulness in solving practical problems'. Initially, the practical use to which the results of Flanagan's study were put was in the selection of suitable candidates for aircraft training. Candidates were presented with simulated critical incidents and their aptitude for coping with and controlling the 'incidents' was observed and analysed.

In this present study the subject population (the one nurse in charge of the theatre or ward during a routine list) would be coping with and controlling real 'critical incidents' in the work situation. What constituted a real critical incident would be the decision of the individual nurse involved. The perception of critical elements in the work situation, both of a stressful and satisfactory nature, is very much an individual experience; this was demonstrated not only in the pre-pilot study discussed later in this chapter but also in the main study, during which there were one or two outstanding examples.

Having considered the type of information required for the study, satisfactory and stressful incidents considered outstanding or critical by the individual concerned, the decision next to be taken was how to collect the information. A form was constructed which was felt to be suitable for use in the pre-pilot study. There was space for three comments and space for the appropriate place on the rating scale to be marked (appendix II). This tool proved unsuitable immediately it was tried out as it was far too structured. As many nurses have done when testing theories of documentation, such as while working with the nursing process (Heath and Law, 1982), the researcher reverted at once to a plain piece of paper for the recording of the information. This created the required flexibility for the collection of the variety and amount of information produced by the informal interviews at the end of each session. The final version of this recording system formed the last three pages of the research tool (appendix III). Interviews are known to produce large amounts of information (Polit and Hungler, 1978) and this was found to be the case in the present study. It was necessary to categorise the large amount and variety of information, and three broad categories of comment emerged during these interview sessions. It was discovered that the comments about the work situation were either to do with patients, with colleagues or with the adminstration of the situation. On no occasion in the pre-pilot study (or the main study) were personal reasons for stress or satisfaction introduced into the informal discussions during the interview.

Table 2 shows how these three broad categories of comment

Table 2 Categories of perceived incidents and intensity of incident experience recorded at interview, and decribed as the subject variables

Theatre, satisfying incidents	Ward, satisfying incidents
patient-centred	patient-centred
staff-centred	staff-centred
administration-centred	administration-centred
Theatre, satisfaction intensity	Ward, satisfaction intensity
patient-centred	patient-centred
staff-centred	staff-centred
administration-centred	administration-centred
Theatre, stressful incidents	Ward, stressful incidents
patient-centred	patient-centred
staff-centred	staff-centred
administration-centred	administration-centred
Theatre, stress intensity	Ward, stress intensity
patient-centred	patient-centred
staff-centred	staff-centred
administration-centred	administration-centred

(patient-centred, staff-centred and administration-centred) made the 24 subjective variables used in this study.

At the beginning of the pre-pilot study the research tool consisted of three pages for recording information, one of which was a check-list of environmental and organisational items (presence of windows, number of staff and so forth) and the other two of which were for recording the interview comments from the theatre and ward staff (see appendix II). By the fourth day the final version had evolved (see appendix III) and this was used on the fifth and last day of the pre-pilot study. The major alterations, apart from the additions to the check-list, were concerned with the information-collecting techniques. The information from the nursing staff interviews required a much freer format for recording than was realised initially, and the environmental and organisational information-collection was discovered to be suited to a more formal collection arrangement. It was also decided that anecdotal information given freely at interview would be recorded. Although it could not form part of the analysis, it did provide an understanding of the whole scenario.

The morning and afternoon sessions of the final day of the pre-pilot study saw the use of the completed research tool and produced extremely rewarding though, as was subsequently found, somewhat atypical observation recordings. The morning in the theatre had been 'bad'; that is, stress was experienced and observed to be experienced. No surgery had taken place until two hours after the booked start although preparations for a major thoracic operating list had been completed at the stated time. The preoperative signing of the consent form had been omitted and the patient lay anaesthetised while the problem was resolved.

What resulted from this difficulty was that the start of the afternoon list was considerably delayed and involved cancellations of patients, changes of mind from the doctors and premedication being given at inappropriate times or not at all. There was even one patient who turned up unexpectedly on the ward having bypassed the normal admission system, as his consultant had given him his operation date during an out-patient visit and had informed no-one else.

The researcher, that is, myself, in the role of non-participant observer, experienced intense anxiety on behalf of the nursing staff both in the theatre and on the ward, but what unfolded from this day's events illustrated that my perceptions of stressful and satisfactory events were not necessarily the same as those of the nurses involved in the situation. The experiences of the day were collected together in the late afternoon and the results from the theatre and the ward produced the following.

1. *In the operating theatre* Although the staff had been under pressure brought about by the delayed start under the competent leadership of the young nurse in charge (state enrolled nurse) they had coped cheerfully and competently. Table 3 shows the five acknowledged areas of stress, the intensity of that stress as indicated on the 1–5 rating scale and the category of stress to which each belonged, either patient-, staff- or administration-centred.

2. *On the ward* The ward, which was a large full 'Nightingale' ward, presented such a calm and ordered appearance when I arrived to interview the nurse in charge (the ward sister) that it hardly seemed possible that it could be an area experiencing any organisational difficulties. This ward had had the care of the patients due for surgery on the afternoon list, a list delayed by problems occurring during the morning list. Certainly the incidents assumed to be stressful were reflected by the sister's recognition of them and their intensity, as is shown in table 4.

The total stress score for the ward was 18, but what was interesting was the satisfaction score of this nurse in charge, which

Table 3 Perceived stress experience, with scores (theatre)

Comment	Score
One sister was off sick	2
The only experienced staff nurse was on holiday	4
All learners were new that day	5
The only porter was at a trade union meeting (he returned in time to transport the next patient)	3
The staff were worrying about the effect that the morning list problems would have on afternoon operating list	2
Total score	16

Table 4 Perceived stress experience, with scores (ward)

Comment	Score
The patient third on the list had had no premedication as the order of the list had been changed three times	5
A patient arrived who was not on the operating list, but who had been added because of his extreme anxiety	5
There were two patients sleeping off their premedications who were (hopefully) for surgery the following day	5
The 'day case' had been sent home, and later it was stated that he need not have been	1
There was general awareness of mix up and confusion over cancellations	2
Total score	18

highlighted the manner in which the satisfactions of the day had offset the difficulties encountered. The satisfaction score was 28, and table 5 shows what contributed to this. 'The ward was full' perhaps needs a little explanation. When the ward was 'full' there could be no unexpected admissions. Therefore, every bed being occupied did relieve anxiety.

It was this set of observations from the final session of the pre-pilot study which indicated the possible existence of a relationship between high satisfaction scores and perception of stress, and the reverse, and it was decided therefore to include in the analysis a

Table 5 Perceived satisfaction experience, with scores (ward)

Comment	Score
The ward itself, although full, was quiet. Sister had done most of the stocktaking and some teaching	4
There were sufficient senior staff to do the nursing	5
A successful expedition to the airport for a patient who had had both legs amputated	5
There had been no deaths, whereas the previous weeks deaths had occurred daily	5
The patients had been able to sleep as the ward was quiet	5
The ward was full	4
Total score	**28**

correlation of high scores for satisfaction and low scores for stress, and vice versa. These observations were also felt to demonstrate the validity of the research tool in relation to the study. The research tool appeared to collect the desired information and also to 'protect' it from observer influence. Hopefully, when the information was subjected to statistical analysis it might reasonably be expected to yield logical results.

10 Collection of information

The information for the main study was collected and recorded during one four-week period, each week covering the five days Monday to Friday. This provided for a maximum of forty routine sessions, twenty morning and twenty afternoon. An all-day session was counted as one session although it consisted of one morning and one afternoon session. No session was missed. Each week of information collecting took place within a different area health authority. The one routine operating list observed could be in any of the theatres within a theatre suite or, should the area health authority's work organisation involve more than one hospital, in any one of the theatres of those hospitals. The nurse in charge of the ward or wards, having the care of the patients operated on during the one routine list observed, would be interviewed in the same way as the nurse in charge of the running of that list in the operating theatre. The research tool allowed the information to be collected in a manner suitable for computer analysis (see appendix III) and, at the end of each week, the data recorded from the observations and interviews was sent to be card-punched.

Because of the type of observer/observed relationship used in this study the use of the research tool was freely discussed with the nurse in charge and others in the operating theatre, including those consultant anaesthetic and surgical staff who were interested in the study. The noting of information on a form is likely to produce a considerable amount of anxiety in those observed and the introduction of any additional stress element into the work situation needed to be avoided. This open approach appeared to have the desired effect in that anxiety about a non-team member appeared to be minimal. One of the questions put during the unstructured, though probing, interviews concerned any anxiety experienced because of

59

the observer's (my) presence. Only one nurse in charge (a sister) admitted to any feeling at all but said that this had been more of an awareness of someone different in the operating theatre than any-thing else and that even this had disappeared within the first 10 minutes. Most staff mentioned that they were so used to different people being in the operating theatre in addition to the actual oper-ating team – people such as learners and observers from the various hospital departments, and visiting senior staff – that my presence had just been part of the usual environment. Certainly, these remarks were confirmed by the observed presence of a number of different 'others' in operating theatres during the routine lists and this could well be an environmental element to include in further study. The theatre in which the sister worked who mentioned the sensation of awareness was not an area having frequent visitors. There were frequent and unprompted comments, though, that indicated the presence of some behaviour modification among staff, both nurses and doctors. These statements were remarks such as, 'We know all about stress here – you've come to the right place' or 'It's all gone so smoothly today but that's because you're here and everyone is on their best behaviour'.

Those occasions when the observer was seen as a threat tended to be during the interview sessions, which took place outside the im-mediate work area, in the rest room or office, and which might well have been seen by other staff as a far more private method of col-lecting information than the noting of items on a form. Several interviews were ended effectively by short comments from senior nursing staff like 'Still here?' or 'Not finished yet?', which made both the interviewee and interviewer feel guilty about wasting time. One nursing officer was most specific on one occasion before the interview, saying to me, 'Don't make what you're doing sound too interesting – I want to keep sister here, not going off to university'.

There were several occasions during which the role of non-partici-pant observer was difficult to maintain and the experience of stress was mine rather than anyone else's. While the recording of such episodes is really outside the parameters of this study they are probably very relevant to the quality of patient care received, and also provide a possible indication of the presence of nursing staff defence mechanisms (Menzies, 1970) which can prevent recog-nition of patient anxiety and stress. In a more complete study about the presence of stress in operating theatres some form of measure-ment of quality of patient care received would be of value, for the indications appeared to be that in those areas where stress was highest in this study (H2) quality of care left a great deal to be desired. The following examples serve to illustrate this point.

One of the more striking incidents concerning quality of patient care received occurred during a situation that demonstrated clearly that the perception of what did or did not constitute a critical incident was very much an individual experience. On this occasion a cholecystectomy with operative cholangiogram was being performed during a routine morning list of reasonable size (that is, there were three patients for elective surgical procedures, obviously planned to be comfortably within the experience of the surgical registrar performing the operations). A staff nurse was the nurse in charge and scrubbed for each case. As this operation proceeded and the moment arrived at which the X-ray would need to be taken no move was made to inform the X-ray department staff who, knowing that such a case was being performed, would be awaiting (and indeed were awaiting) the instruction to come to theatre. The appropriate flexible cannula was inserted, the radio-opaque solution prepared, and this was followed by the inevitable query 'Where's X-ray' from the surgeon. The stress experienced by myself (who had worked 15 years as a sister in operating theatres) was so intense that withdrawal offered the only relief. The incident was completely ignored by the staff nurse taking the case. Not only was it not worthy of mention during the subsequent interview but also the mere acknowledgement that a delay had occurred (and had caused the patient to have at least 25 minutes longer than necessary under the anaesthetic) had to be dragged out by direct questioning. This could not be recorded as a stress for it had not been perceived as a stressful incident, but it does give pause for thought.

On another occasion I was present during an out-patient session where all the patients had had short general anaesthetics. The procedures and small operations were such cases as cystoscopies, examinations under anaesthetic and one vasectomy in a young man about to marry who belonged to a family with a history of a hereditary degenerative disease. This list, in fact, from the patients' viewpoint was very stressful for several of the ladies present had most tragic personal circumstances. (This information had been given to me directly by the consultant, who was particularly interested in my study of stress.) The list was well-organised and unhurried and, when all was completed, I went through to the small and well-equipped recovery area in which the morning's patients were gradually waking up, apparently comfortably, under the care of a pleasant and cheerful staff nurse. I then realised that two of the patients were weeping quietly and, partly stepping outside the non-participant role, drew the attention of the staff nurse to this. 'Oh, they often cry after an anaesthetic' was the brisk and cheerful smiling response. No stresses were acknowledged as having been perceived by the staff nurse who remained pleasant and cheerful throughout and had ignored the episodes (and my interference in drawing atttention to such things and actually sitting with each patient for a time).

On the more positive side there were also outstanding examples of high quality of care, the most interesting one being provided by a recovery ward in the third hospital visited. As with the incident just related, the activity of this area was geared to the needs of those patients having short general anaesthetics for the type of procedure or surgery that requires admission for the day or part of the day. The recovery ward was spacious and the patients were at various stages of postoperative recovery, either sleeping, dozing propped up on a few pillows or even sitting up having tea and sandwiches. The tea trolley had a prominent place in the ward recovery activity and the sister in charge and myself had a good discussion about the fierce hunger experienced by many patients following short procedures and short general anaesthetics, and the faintness and nausea that will result if this want is not recognised and relieved. The quality of whole patient care in this area was outstanding when viewed from the context of the whole study and, should further study be undertaken concerning stress in these acute areas, some indication of quality of care must certainly be included because, and this is more fully discussed in the following chapters, the hospital in which the two incidents causing the observer stress occurred was also the one that had the highest stress and lowest satisfaction scores.

This chapter is intended to provide an overall impression of the data collection, some of the experiences of the observer, and the possible need for quality of care indications should any further study be undertaken.

Part III: The analysis

11 Preliminary organisation of information

The collection and organisation of the information forming the environmental variables was straightforward. This information was collected from the operating theatres only during the routine operating sessions. Once the final selection of items had been tested during the pre-pilot study the collection of information was simply a matter of recording, on the appropriate page of the research tool (appendix III), the presence or absence of certain environmental and administrative items. The items included on this final list, which is not considered to be an exhaustive one, were a selection of those mentioned in the available relevant literature as contributing to stress, those recognised in a general way by nurses as being sources of anxiety (meal-break organisation comes into this category) and those that could be noted by one person during the working-through of a routine operating list (see appendix III). This information was intended to provide the background against which the perceived stress or satisfaction experience of the nurse in charge would be considered.

This numerical information was basic and quantitative, merely establishing the background detail, but even so it allowed for some interesting comparisons before statistical inferences were considered. For instance, in table 6 some of the basic operating list information is recorded for hospitals H1, H2, H3 and H4. Similarities and differences are immediately apparent, the most notable differences being recorded for H2. This operating theatre had, in this study, the highest number of schedule alterations (36) during its one five-day period of routine operating and the highest number of alterations on any one routine list (22). Bear in mind when

Table 6 Comparison of operating list information by hospital

Operating list information	H1	H2	H3	H4
Number of morning sessions recorded	5	4	5	4
Number of afternoon sessions recorded	5	4	5	4
Number of all-day sessions recorded	0	1	0	1
Premedication time control	A	A	A	A
Operation time control	S	S	S	S
Total number of routine operations recorded Monday to Friday	65	51	55	39
Total number of alterations recorded Monday to Friday	15	36	13	7
Highest number of alterations on one list	1	22	3	3
Number of lists without any alterations	5	3	4	6

A = Anaesthetist
S = Sister

looking at these figures that none of the operating lists observed were interrupted by emergency, unplanned surgery. It is also interesting to look at the similarities between hospitals. The surgeon controls the numbers and types of patients for surgery as well as the patients' positions on the list. Two other significant members of the operating theatre staff 'control' the time elements in each patient's case: the anaesthetist controls the premedication time and the sister controls the overall management time. It hardly needs a research study to recognise the sort of pressure that 22 changes to one four-hour routine list will produce for these other significant members of staff in the operating theatre in order to maintain the care, well-being and safety of the patients concerned.

The full list of variables, not all of which were amenable to this form of tabular investigation using the preliminary computer analysis results, is given in appendix IV.

The collection of information providing the subjective variables for this study was also straightforward. The interviews in both the theatres and the wards opened with a few explanatory remarks to the effect that the research was intended to support otherwise tentative hypotheses relating to stress in qualified nurses on the day of a patient's operation. This was followed by a question as to

whether or not the observer's presence had presented any problems. Then came the questions as to what had been good or
difficult about the session. This approach was successful in producing a large amount of information, much larger than had been
anticipated, a recognised interview phenomenon (Sweeney and
Olivieri, 1981). The question that completed the interview and
rounded it off concerned outstanding, good or difficult incidents
occurring within the past six weeks. It was thought that this information, which would not be used in the computer analysis, could
well provide a meaningful background to the whole study.
appendix V contains a selection of nurse comments, including these
anecdotal ones.

A total of 80 interviews were conducted, 40 in the operating
theatres and 40 on the ward. There was a response rate of 100% for,
although all the nurses were asked if they would prefer to withdraw, they all agreed to be interviewed. As had been discovered
during the pre-pilot study, the staff comments could be categorised
into the same three areas, namely, those in which the patient had
contributed to the experience of the nurse in charge, those in which
staff-related concerns were emphasised and those in which the
administration of the day had prompted the comment. These
comments were made quite freely.

Both the collection of information concerning the comments
made about different experiences of the day and the intensity of the
individual nurse's experience were required. It was intended that
this approach would provide a balance between the (presupposed)
greater number of administrative pressures of a less stressful nature
than the one or two patient-related stresses, assumed to be more
intense. (The underlying assumptions in this study are addressed
in chapter 6).

A few comments were made which might be placed in more than
one category. These remarks were usually those concerned with the
number and experience of nursing staff and the organisation of the
meal breaks. It is perhaps of interest to note here that none of the 80
interviews contained any comment about personal outside stresses
or worries, a point that would appear to raise a great many questions in view of the vast body of literature describing the variety of
life stresses today. This could, of course, be the result of the type of
interview conducted but, although there was open recognition of
personnel incompatibilities, both nurse/nurse and doctor/nurse,
there was no hint that public transport difficulties, flat car tyres or

other personal problems of any sort might influence the pressure of the day's experience.

While the information collected was being card-punched in readiness for the detailed computer analysis, a preliminary manual analysis of the comments made during the 80 interviews was conducted. It was expected that this would provide some indication of the overall results. Table 7 is a comparison by hospital of the number of stressful and satisfactory incidents identified by the nurses interviewed.

Table 7 Comparison of the number and category of incidents identified during nurse interviews, by hospital

	Theatre						Ward					
	Patient		Staff		Admin		Patient		Staff		Admin	
	−	+	−	+	−	+	−	+	−	+	−	+
H1	2	9	4	9	2	10	3	8	3	9	4	8
H2	0	8	14	8	4	5	9	3	5	11	12	6
H3	0	6	15	14	6	7	4	7	2	17	10	15
H4	5	7	6	10	5	8	1	8	2	8	6	8
Total	7	30	39	41	17	30	17	26	12	45	32	37
Grand total	Stress(−)54:Satisfactory(+)101						Stress(−)61:Satisfactory(+)98					

The information in table 2 would appear to support those who state that satisfaction is as great, if not greater, a part of the experience of the working day in hospital as is stress (Nichols et al, 1981), for the overall ratio of satisfaction to stress in number of incidents recorded is about 2 : 1. The staff-related experiences in both areas appear to be the more frequently recognised, particularly for satisfaction. This suggests the presence of the strong supportive groups within nursing (Menzies, 1970).

Hospital H2 indicates a somewhat negative patient approach on the wards (9 incidents) and possibly a non-supportive, negative attitude between colleagues in the operating theatres (14). H3 shows a similar high number of staff-related incidents on the negative side (15) but it is suggested that the almost identical number of staff satisfaction comments balances this. Organisational or administrative stresses also attract more recognition in the wards of H2 and H3.

The intensity scores for each of the 40 sessions were totalled. The

Table 8 Comparison of highest scoring session in each experience category

	Theatre		Ward	
	Stress	Satisfaction	Stress	Satisfaction
Patient-related score	3	4	12	5
Staff-related score	4	6	4	17
Administration-related score	16	5	16	6

nurse concerned judged the intensity of the incident identified as stressful or satisfying by the use of a rating scale, numbered 1 to 5, with 1 scoring low. There was no upper limit set to the number of incidents that the nurse might identify. Table 8 is a comparison of the highest scoring session in each category of comment made at interview.

What is felt to be of interest here, and of possible management implication, is the almost identical stress and satisfaction intensity pattern in both wards and theatres for administrative experience. In table 7 (above) the number of negative administrative theatre comments totals 17, and in the wards 32. Perhaps it might be inferred, from considering these totals in relation to the figures for the highest scoring session, that administrative and organisational anxieties in the operating theatre during routine operating lists are more intense than those in the ward, but that there are more of them on the wards. One of the underlying assumptions of this study was that administrative stress might be more frequent but of lesser intensity. It is suggested that this would appear to be the case. A further underlying assumption was that it was expected to find few patient-related stresses for, after all, the surgical team is trained to care for patients undergoing surgery, but that the intensity of the stress experience that did occur would be high. In the theatres only 7 stress incidents all told were mentioned and the highest intensity scores were also low, being 3 (table 9). The wards experienced far more stress-related incidents (17) and had the highest intensity score for any one session (12).

There are several possible reasons for these differences in perception or experience. The first may well be related to the fact that ward staff feel less well supported than theatre staff or that, with the use of recovery rooms, postoperative care skills are not required as much as formerly. As in all studies the information

Table 9 Comparison of intensity range for each comment category.

	Theatre		Ward	
	Stress	Satisfaction	Stress	Satisfaction
Patient-related intensity range	2−3	1−4	3−5	2−5
Staff-related intensity range	1−4	2−5	1−5	1−4
Administration-related intensity range	1−5	1−5	1−5	1−5

gathered raises as many questions as it answers. But, whatever the reasons for the differences here between ward and theatre nurses, the patient-related stress measurement was significant for theatre nurses $p<0.01$ indicating perhaps that, in spite of their concealing or containing obvious stress responses, stress was experienced in the possibly trivial staff-related or administration-related responses.

In this chapter the information collected by direct observation and recording in the operating theatre, and by interview in the theatres and the relevant wards, has been considered briefly. The intention has been to create an overall picture of the ward and theatre situation during routine operating sessions in order to provide a meaningful background for the results of the computer analysis by introducing and using some minimal as well as ordinal measurements (Polit and Hungler, 1978; Rowntree, 1981; Phillips, 1981).

12 Discussion of significant results

This study into aspects of stress in nurses working in operating theatres and the supporting wards produced 14 significant results, 8 of which related to stress. A detailed consideration of all the 38 independent objective variables, and whether or not they were found to have significant influence in terms of perception of stress or satisfaction in individual nurses, is presented in appendix IV. This chapter considers the implications of the 8 significant stress-related results, one of which was the newly-identified variable, the computed 'overrun/underrun' time.

The significance of a result is described in terms of the probability of such a result occurring by chance (that is, influenced by differences in the group being studied, the sample, rather than by an identified variable, such as absence of windows). The probability against such a result occurring by chance is described by using the convention of a measurement lying between 0 and 1, often used with a symbol to indicate 'less than' ($<$) or 'greater than' ($>$). In this study a probability lying between $p<0.5$ and $p>0.01$ was considered to be 'significant' and one lying between $p<0.01$ and $p>0.001$ was considered to be 'highly significant'.

The significance, as used in research, is that concept which allows for the differences in sample populations to be controlled by the identification, measurement and use of these differences in the rejection or acceptance of the hypothesis (Rowntree, 1981). The value of the significance lies in its inherent ability to strengthen conclusions drawn from sample populations that are (possibly) to be applied to target populations. In this study the sample population was, of course, the qualified nurses in the operating theatres and wards having the responsibility for the care of the patient on the day of operation in the selected health authorities (H1, H2, H3, H4). The target population was seen as being all qualified nurses similarly placed in the health authorities of the UK.

The computer programme 'Statistical Package for the Social Sciences' (SPSS) was used. This package is specifically designed to compute the sort of non-parameter data that this study generated, and the study data input at weekly intervals during the four-week data collection period produced a very large amount of information. The volume of descriptive statistics, the sheer numbers of means, modes, medians and standard deviations relating to all the study variables (both the objective, independent ones, and the subjective, dependent ones) would have been impossible to deal with by hand. Various computerised statistical tests, tests dealing with differences between samples, relationships, ranking and small numbers were used (descriptions of the tests are in appendix VI) and 8 significant stress results identified (table 10). These 8 stress results, 5 of which fall into the 'highly significant' category and 3 into the 'significant' category, are summarised in table 5.

Table 10 Summary of significant stress findings

Area	Cause	Probability
Theatre	Temperature perceived as hot	$p < 0.001$
Theatre	List inaccuracies	$p < 0.005$
Ward	Overrun/underrun time	$p < 0.005$
Theatre	Absence of windows	$p < 0.007$
Theatre	Meal breaks	$p < 0.007$
Theatre	Patient crisis	$p < 0.01$
Theatre	Presence of theatre-experienced staff	$p < 0.03$
Theatre	Observed stress	$p < 0.03$

A final, brief look at these results shows that there is only one 'ward' stress here, the new variable, the computed 'overrun/ underrun'time. It is suggested that the appearance of only one ward stress is a function of the research design in that any new variables identified could only be those influencing the theatre or the theatre and ward together, but not the ward alone as the observations were made only in the theatre.

Another immediately noticeable stress result is that the patient-crisis variable registered as a significant stress result. Bear in mind that during the interview the nurse did not by any means say 'patient crisis' (if one had occurred) when asked about the good and bad experiences of the day. There were, in observable objective terms, very few 'patient crises' in this study perceived to be so by the nurse (and some others that did occur were only stressful to myself as the observer). It was interesting, therefore, to identify such a significant measurement of its influence as a variable in this study. It is not of course an unexpected stress given the nature of the work in the area being studied. What was found in the results which was unexpected was the number of management elements having a highly significant influence upon the stress perceptions of the day. List inaccuracies, the overrun/underrun time, meal breaks and skill mix are all management areas. That these should be causing a significant measure of stress experience in qualified nurses is cause for concern.

A more detailed consideration of all significant variables now follows.

STRESS-RELATED RESULTS

Perception of theatre temperature

There was a highly significant correlation found between the perception of temperature as hot by the scrubbed personnel and their stress scores $p < 0.001$. A feeling of 'being hot' is a difficulty encountered by the scrubbed personnel, surgical and nursing, and can be observed directly when the staff are under pressure. Improved ventilation and lighting have lessened this problem to a certain extent. This was one of the improvements that led to the loss of windows in operating theatres.

The range of temperatures was found to be 19°C to 28°C, 75% of the theatres having temperatures of 23°C or below, and 22°C being the mode (14 sessions). 21°–22°C is the usual recommended temperature (Brigden, 1974) but this may well be higher on those occasions when the very young or very old are having surgery. The highest temperature, 28°C, was recorded in a theatre that had an air conditioning failure and although the scrubbed personnel were very uncomfortable they were also very philosophical about the situation.

Inaccuracies in the list

A significant relationship between staff stress and list inaccuracies was established, as had been expected. In this study 2.5% of all list alterations were because of some inaccuracy, and the significance between the perception of staff-related stress incidents and inaccuracies was found to be $p<0.005$.

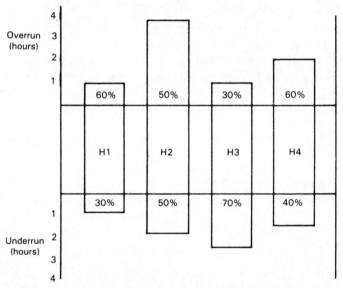

Maximum overrun time was 230 minutes, maximum underrun time 150 minutes
NB Hospital H1 had 10% of lists completed on time

Figure 5   The overrun/underrun time by hospital, demonstrating the percentage of lists over- and underrunning in each case

Overrun/underrun time

A time consideration was computed which was the difference between the time allowed and the time taken for the list (see research tool, appendix III). The study indicated that this is an area of enormous variability for the time range encompassed 380 minutes, from minus 150 minutes to plus 230 minutes. Figure 5 shows in diagrammatic form the percentage of lists affected and the maximum time noted by hospital. Only one hospital (H1) had any lists finishing on time (on time being 15 minutes either way) and, although H1 had 60% overrunning and 30% underrunning, the time involved was never more than an hour. The other hospitals present a wide range of time variations, the most notable ones being H2, having 50% of lists overrunning, with a maximum time of 4 hours late, and H3, having 70% of lists underrunning, with a maximum time of 2½ hours early. The overall percentages for overrun/underrun, the study total, are:

- 50% of all lists overran;
- 47.5% of all lists underran;
- 2.5% of all lists finished on time (H1 only).

There are certainly implications in this result not only for staff stress but also for the efficient use of manpower, equipment and premises. It has to be emphasised that these times are for routine lists only, measured over one five-day period in each hospital. Emergency surgery did not at any time interrupt these sessions of planned elective surgery.

Interestingly, it was only the ward staff who showed a significant stress relationship between the overrun/underrun time and the staff-related incidents, with a probability of $p<0.005$.

One reason for theatre staff registering no significance here could well be the disappearance (almost) of their meal break from the organisation of the day, which would lessen the time pressures between operating sessions. The Lewin Report (Department of Health and Social Security, 1970) in particular mentions the necessity for the theatre environment to be cleaned and 'rested' between the morning and afternoon sessions. This time should be amenable to meal-break planning, but this is rarely the case.

The underrun/overrun time was an acknowledged stress. Ward staff frequently voiced worries about premedication timings. In H3, the hospital registering the greatest underuse of time, one ward nurse in charge (a sister) said at interview that she would never cease to be thankful for the appointment of a new anaesthetic consultant who favoured the use of oral premedications. These were given as prescribed to all the patients for surgery before the list started and then whatever 'they' did ('they' being the surgeons in the operating theatre) the patients were safe and comfortable. A selection of comments from the interviews and the anecdotes will be found in appendix V.

Presence/absence of windows

In this study there was found to be a significant relationship between the absence of windows and stress scores in theatre nursing staff, from $p>0.04$ to $p<0.007$ (see appendix IV). A 'window' was considered as such when it was of plain glass with a horizon. Frosted glass was not considered a window. The windows varied in type and placing; some overlooked the theatre service corridor which had windows to the outside, some were vertical or high horizontal 'slits', double glazed, that look straight out. Interestingly, the presence or absence of windows did not feature to any extent in the comments apart from the odd remark that a certain theatre was 'nice and light'.

In this study 57.5% of operating theatres were windowless and the significant measurement relating to their absence and staff-centred stress incidents was found to be $p<0.0065$, with the relationship between their absence and staff perception of intensity significant at $p<0.01$. The relationship between presence or absence of windows and the effect on staff attracts some ambivalence as the literature review in the study records, so it is of particular interest and relevance to have such a positive result.

Meal breaks

The management of the staff meal break and the difficulty this attracted featured in about a quarter of the interviews. The 'mix' of staff was seen as adding to nurse difficulties. The learners were the members of staff to have regular meal breaks which contributed to the 72.5% of meal breaks taken properly. There was frequently observed pressure upon nurses responsible for the organising of meal breaks, particularly if the afternoon session belonged to a different consultant. The meal-break management in this study (which concerned lunch breaks as the routine lists as anticipated occurred during the prime shift hours) was observed to have 2.5% missed completely, 25.0% interrupted and 72.5% taken properly.

There was a relationship between the stress scores of theatre nursing staff and meal breaks, found to be significant in the following three category areas:

- patient-centred stress incident, significant at $p<0.007$;
- patient-centred stress intensity, significant at $p<0.004$;
- administrative-stress incidents, significant at $p<0.04$.

Patient crisis

The patient crises in this study tended to be anxieties concerning the frailty of a particular patient and cancellations of operations (particularly those concerning the elderly who had had successive days of preoperative starvation, and with heavier bleeding than 'normal' during surgery) rather than cardiac or respiratory arrest. A significant probability result was discovered between the stress in the theatre nursing staff and the occurrence of a patient crisis, $p<0.01$. A patient crisis of some sort was experienced in 12.5% of all the observed operating lists.

The only intense patient crisis observed was one that occurred during the pre-pilot study when a patient had a respiratory collapse and had to be resuscitated by the nursing staff. It happened during the lunchtime meal break and change-over of operating teams, and there was no recovery room. This was perceived as an intense satisfaction by the nursing staff who had had the care of this patient at his moment of need, but as a worry and anxiety to the ward staff who received him back to bed, for they were short-staffed, were mainly junior staff (no sister on duty) and the ward was large and open-plan.

Number of theatre-experienced qualified nursing staff

A significant relationship was found to exist between the presence of theatre-experienced qualified staff and stress ($p<0.03$) which was surprising as it is thought that to have nurses with the required specialist experience could only be a satisfaction.

It is suggested that perhaps, whereas it is a relief to have qualified nursing support in the operating theatre for the scrubbed nurse, there is a possible ambivalence where theatre-experienced staff are concerned. One theatre sister said during interview that she found the presence of the experienced clinical teacher a strain. She knew that the clinical teacher's interest was focused on the learners but felt that she was constantly under review as well. It appeared from the figures in this study that two or three theatre-experienced nursing staff were usual (75% of all sessions) but there was one occasion (2.5% of total sessions) when there was no theatre-experienced qualified nurse present. The overall breakdown of theatre-experienced qualified nurses present was found to be:

- no such nurse present at 1 session;

- 1 such nurse present at 7 sessions;
- 2 such nurses present at 16 sessions;
- 3 such nurses present at 14 sessions;
- 4 such nurses present at 2 sessions.

There were 6 items relating to number and type of theatre staff and 2 relating to what was expected of them (on call, staying late). Learner nurses, mentioned as a source of stress during the interviews, were sometimes not present (study range 0–4 for observed sessions) and, although this was an area that looked as though a significant stress level might emerge, when the figures were subjected to a Fisher's Exact Test (appendix VI), a test for small figures, no significance was found. As the range for theatre-experienced qualified nurses was also 0–4 and that for qualified nurses 2–4, perhaps the significant results in this area should be interpreted with caution as all of the actual numbers are small. As significant results have emerged this could be one area in which a study of stress experience, satisfaction experience and optimum numbers and quality of staff would be of value.

Observed stress

Observed stress in theatre staff was included in the study to act as a possible check on the internal validity of the research. A significant correlation was found to exist between stress observed in the theatre (noted as 'yes' or 'no' for coding) and stress scores in theatre staff, in relation to staff-centred perceived incidents and intensity, $p<0.034$ and $p<0.036$ respectively. These results were felt to be some validation of the research study which could be of value when considering the results, particularly those that were considered by the observer to be unexpected.

Type of session

Sessions were of three types: morning (45%), afternoon (42.5%) and all day (12.5%). The type of session being worked produced a significant satisfaction correlation in the scores of theatre nursing staff, the measurement being $p<0.03$. It would have been useful to relate this satisfaction indicator to specific sessions, particularly those indicating meal-break pressures but with the size of the study this was not possible. In view of this any interpretation must be approached with caution. Certainly it would appear to be generally recognised and mentioned during the interview sessions that the all-day session with one surgical team (of which there were two in this study) produced far fewer management or organisational pressures in the operating theatre. When time on a morning list is out of control and overrunning, anxiety in anaesthetic staff, as well as recovery staff, can reach very high levels contributing to the observed stress noted in this study. In this study, however, there were no unpleasant scenes observed between surgeons competing for the same resources of manpower, time and equipment (perhaps because there was an observer).

Staff expected to stay late

A high proportion (87.5%) of the nurses working in the operating theatre were expected to stay late, that is, work longer than the allotted time. This was found to be related at a significant level with satisfaction scores in theatre nursing staff in both patient-centred and administration-centred remarks, at $p<0.03$ and $p<0.04$ respectively. Although the figure of 87.5% was not unexpected in view of the use of time demonstrated in the overrun/underrun time, it was a surprise that satisfaction was the experience of the day that registered in this study, for staff did mention during the interview sessions the problem of repeatedly finishing late. It is possible that other factors influenced this result, possibly overtime payments, but it is more likely that the time pressure was 'removed' by the 'expected to stay late' acceptance.

The cost implications of such a high proportion of staff being expected to work late would be interesting to follow up in a future study, particularly in relation to the use of the 37½-hour working week and the optimum number of staff for each routine list.

Number of qualified staff

The number and type of nurse and a 'good mix' were important factors for the nurse in charge of theatre lists. For example, about 12.5% of the 'satisfaction' comments related to the 'good mix'. A significant correlation was found between presence of qualified staff and the perceived satisfactory administration elements of the day, at $p<0.05$. Two qualified nurses were present for two-thirds of all observed lists and three or more were present during the other one-third.

Learners tended to be seen as a strain though this did not register as a significance, probably due to the small group numbers. 'Well, if you really want to know, the best list we've had recently was six weeks ago when there were no learners of any sort – medical, nursing or operating department assistants – in the theatre,' was the comment made by one nurse. Too many sisters could also present problems but it was suspected that this was possibly related to interpersonal or professional problems rather than number or type of staff present.

The number of qualified staff for each session was found to be:

- 2 qualified nurses for 67.5% of all observed sessions;
- 3 qualified nurses for 27.5% of all observed sessions;
- 4 qualified nurses for 5.0% of all observed sessions.

SATISFACTION-RELATED RESULTS

List additions

Thirty per cent of alterations to operating lists were found to be additions. Perhaps, surprisingly, this did not feature as a stress at all in the analysis; instead there was found to be a significant relationship with staff perception of satisfactory events in the theatre, significant at $p<0.005$. It is suggested that this has support from the relatively high number of occasions (75%) on which there was mention of patient-related satisfaction experience within the operating theatre. It might also be assumed that the overrun time is so common (see Figure 5 above) that, if it is not excessive, it is accepted as some sort of 'norm'.

List cancellations

Forty per cent of all alterations to operating lists were cancellations. As with additions a significance of $p<0.005$ was found to exist in the relationship between theatre staff satisfaction, reflected in their patient-centred comments, and cancellations (see appendix V).

The presence or absence of a TSSU

The theatre sterile supply unit (TSSU) produced an unexpected satisfaction correlation with its absence of $p<0.01$. Problems were acknowledged to exist during interviews between these units and the nursing staff requiring their services. At one time nurses ran these units but this is no longer the policy of the hospital services. One hospital in the study still had its theatre sterile supply unit run by the theatre staff (H1, which came out rather better than hospitals 2, 3 and 4 on the mean rank scores for stress and satisfaction, see figures 6–9 below). One comment made in hospital 3 was, 'There is only one person in the TSSU who knows what the pressures are. If you ring for help – and this always seems to happen at lunchtime and he is on his lunch break – you are often left without help because the others do not realise how vital it is to answer a call.' The person in TSSU referred to here had been a member of the theatre team as an orderly for many years prior to his move to the theatre sterile supply unit so understood the essential nature of the work in a theatre. Of all observed sessions in this study, 65% were supplied with their basic sterile requirements of linen, swabs and instruments from a theatre sterile supply unit.

COMPUTED STRESS AND SATISFACTION RELATIONSHIPS

Correlation between stress and satisfaction scores

A correlation between low satisfaction and high stress scores, and high satisfaction and low stress scores, was found in operating theatre staff.

When the incidence of satisfaction was low there was found to be a significant relationship between the number and intensity of stress experiences, significant at $p<0.007$ and $p<0.008$ respectively. The reverse was also true but not at such high levels for, when stress incidents and intensity scored low, satisfaction scores were high, the probabilities being $p<0.021$ and $p<0.034$ respectively.

Figures 6–9 (see also figure 1, chapter 1) indicate visually the relationship by hospital of the stress and satisfaction scores in the wards and theatres. The mean rank scores for total satisfaction and stress in wards and theatres of each hospital are used for these calculations. Hospital 2 (H2) demonstrated the lowest satisfaction scores for both wards and theatres and the highest stress for wards. H2, as is shown in table 6 (chapter 11), had the highest number of alterations to its operating lists during the week (36), and the highest for any one list (22). H2 was also the hospital in which the two outstanding examples of nurse failure to recognise patient need were observed.

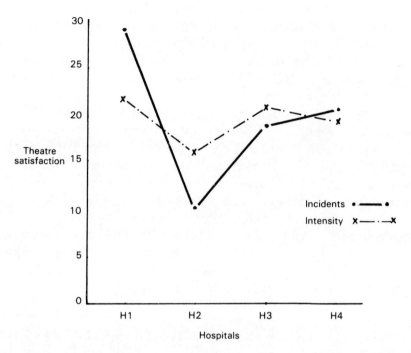

Figure 6   Graph indicating mean rank scores for satisfaction in theatres

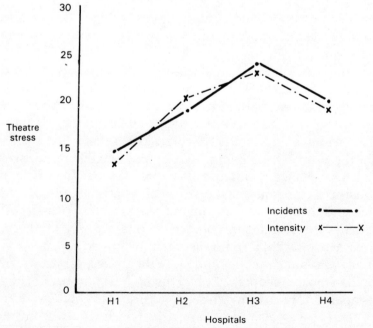

Figure 7   Graph indicating mean rank scores for stress in theatres

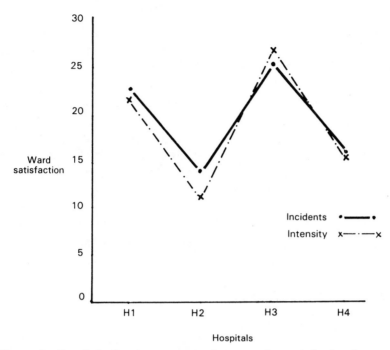

Figure 8 Graph indicating mean rank scores for satisfaction in wards

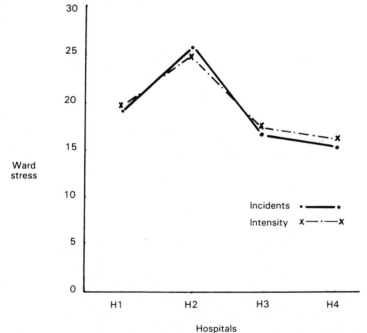

Figure 9 Graph indicating mean rank scores for stress in wards

Reflection of satisfaction between wards and theatres

A correlation was found to exist between the wards and theatres and their separate experience of patient-related and administration satisfactions, at $p<0.032$ and $p<0.017$ respectively.

It is felt that this finding is supported not only by the review of the relevant available literature in which mention is made of satisfaction experience being a large part and usually the greater part of the nursing experience, but also by the preliminary analysis of the comments in which it was demonstrated that remarks concerning satisfaction were consistently higher in all three categories of comment than stress (see table 7).

13 Conclusions, implications and limitations

The two hypotheses explored in this study were (i) that the qualified nurse who is caring for a patient on his day of operation experiences additional stress should a change or changes occur in the expected organisation of the day, and (ii) that there is a relationship between the stress experience of nurses in the wards and the operating theatres. ('Additional', in the context of this study, means over and above the 'expected' pressures and stresses of the day.) It is suggested in this study, which is a first study in this area, that it could perhaps be cautiously implied from the study results that both these hypotheses are upheld, the first somewhat more strongly than the second. The 'not so strong' upholding of the hypothesis may be a function of the overall study design in that the observations could only be undertaken in the operating theatre. The variables 'list inaccuracies' and 'underrun/overrun time' may certainly be described as changes to the expected organisation of the day and the stress experience of nurses associated with these variables had a significance in both cases of $p<0.005$. Again, it must be emphasised that not one of these routine lists observed in the main study was changed because of the need to operate on someone with an emergency or even urgent condition.

The second hypothesis concerning the possible relationship between wards and theatres and the experience of the day is certainly demonstrated to exist in this study (summary table, chapter 1) in H1 and H2, the 'best' and the 'worst' hospitals. This would also appear to be borne out in the significant correlation between the satisfaction scores in ward and theatre areas ($p<0.032$ and $p<0.017$ respectively). But, in the two hospitals not occupying the 'extreme' positions in the comparison of mean rank scores for stress and satisfaction, the position is not so easy to define. However, the correlations between high stress and low satisfaction and high satisfaction and low stress (figures 6–9, chapter 12) are such that cautious support may be suggested for this second hypothesis. What is of interest to note here is that the two outstanding incidents causing extreme anxiety to myself as the observer occurred in H2 (lowest satisfaction and highest stress) went apparently unnoticed by the relevant nurse, and therefore could not feature in the stress or satisfaction perceptions recorded. These incidents, though occurring as they did in the hospital experiencing the highest stress scores, did appear to support the theory that high stress levels in staff adversely affect the quality of care perceived by the patients (Revans, 1972). Although one should not lose sight of the well-supported statement, upheld by both the available literature and by the findings of this study, that satisfaction is as much, if not more, a part of the nurse's experience of the day as is stress, the number of significant management-related stress results found in this study is felt to have implications for nurses and their continuing watch over the quality of their patient care.

IMPLICATIONS OF THE STUDY

The spread of the stress findings was wide within the whole of the environment of the routine operating list, and included stress relating to the patient, to the staff and to certain design and management elements. Certain elements were known to be supported in the available and relevant literature, a case in point being absence of windows. Other elements could well be described as newly-realised, as would appear to be the case with management of meal breaks and the overrun/underrun time.

Several implications for nursing management may be found in the significant stress results listed in table 10 (chapter 12). It was interesting to have a finding recording stress experience in relation to the patient in operating theatre staff because it was felt that the preliminary analysis of the interview comments indicated the presence of strong defence systems (10% of the comments from theatre staff recognised patient-related stress). This could of course have resulted from design weakness in the conduct of the interviews, that is, that their free response allowed the interviewee to select out that which was felt to be irrelevant. But, in spite of this possibility, it is suggested that, although defence systems are present and strong in the nurses, patient-related stresses are stronger. Awareness of this stress is important to nurse managers in their counselling role.

There are several specific implications for nursing management in these stress results. The scarce and expensive manpower and time resources are considered to be the most significant. The stress associated with the overrun/underrun time and the related management of meal breaks can only be a disruptive influence on the staff, as well as being expensive.

The sensible use of scarce resources argues an in-depth understanding of the organisation controlling those resources. Professor Revans' work emphasises time and time again that the understanding of the organisation by all those who work within it will lessen stress and that, in hospitals, this includes doctors as well as nurses.

> 'The critical problems of hospitals are on their wards and in their theatres, and they will be solved only on those wards and in those theatres, they will not be solved elsewhere.' (Revans, 1972)

There are indications also that difficulties could well be expected in relation to the 'mix' of staff in an operating theatre, a problem discussed more fully in chapter 12. The absence of windows as a cause of stress attracted some ambivalence in the literature but in this study was found to be a significant cause of stress. This should help support the case for aware nurses to take an active part in the planning and design stages of new projects.

The correlation between observed and actual stress experience, the feeling of being hot and the stress findings, is probably not very surprising but it is felt to be useful as a possible validation of the research design as a whole.

LIMITATIONS

In a first research study there are bound to be many limitations and some felt to have affected this study are now discussed.

Pre-pilot study

One limitation of this study was felt to be that the hospital used in the pre-pilot study was later realised to be atypical in that the theatres and the supporting wards were built together. Although this one hospital did produce a wide range of type of surgery and type of session it appeared that the relevance of some of the variables to the study itself was not as appropriate as it might have been. For instance, in the pre-pilot study there were no recovery rooms serving any of the operating theatres because the wards were adjacent. The one absolute patient crisis, a respiratory collapse, was observed in these conditions. Recovery rooms are acknowledged to be a service that lessens anxieties for both theatre and ward nursing staff (and anaesthetists), for the recovery room staff are clinical experts in their field and have all the necessities for patient care in the immediate postoperative, postanaesthetic phase readily to hand. No comparisons concerning stress or satisfaction scores could usefully be made in this case as all the theatres in the main study had recovery rooms.

Counting and recording procedures

The counting and recording procedures for swabs, needles and instruments was another area producing a similar difficulty. These procedures differed considerably between hospitals. Some places counted the atraumatic needles and recorded them, some did not. Sometimes the instruments were formally counted by two people, sometimes only the scrub nurse checked the instruments. Swabs were counted in fives, in tens or singly, and could sometimes be counted down into plastic bags when a certain number were 'up'. What was done with this variable was to ascertain the practice in a particular hospital and refer to that as the 'standard'. This meant that 100% of the hospitals were recorded as using a standard counting and recording procedure. Anxiety can be quite acute concerning the counting and recording of items of equipment used during surgery, for the very good reason that such items have to be accounted for before wound closure can safely commence. The joint memorandum 'Safeguards against failure to remove swabs and instruments from patients' (Medical Defence Union and Royal College of Nursing, 1978b) advises on safe practice in this area. It was felt that the variety of systems in use indicated a possible inappropriateness in these counting and recording variables to the requirements of the study. Again, 100% was recorded here for theatres carrying out 'standard procedures'. It was not possible to make comparisons between the counting procedures and the stress or satisfaction scores and, as these were not mentioned in the comments made by staff during the discussions, no general remarks can be made concerning perception of nursing staff about these procedures.

Quality of care indicators

It was felt in retrospect that a simple indication of quality of patient care might have been an advantage. There were outstanding examples of both good and poor care witnessed during this study. Quality of patient care and its possible measurement form a large subject area and are outside the parameters of this present study. H2, which produced both the highest stress levels and the lowest satisfaction levels as indicated on the graphs indicating the mean rank scores, also produced the two incidents described in chapter 10 in which patient stresses went unrecognised by nurses.

Selection of variables

In retrospect it was thought that the criteria for variable selection had not been handled as consistently as they could have been. In the discussion concerning reasons for variable selection in chapter 9 a certain level of information required to be recorded. For instance, patients would be 'numerical', their age and sex would not be recorded. Similarly, operations would be categorised into broad groups (major, intermediate or minor) and would be numbered within those groups. Operating list information went further than this. Alterations were not just counted, different types of alteration were identified as well. There is some ambivalence of feeling concerning the best approach here for, although when the types of information about alterations were analysed collectively there was no significant stress result, when they were analysed separately a significant stress result was identified relating to inaccuracies.

The presence of 'others'

It was during the collecting of the information that the considerable number of 'other' people present during surgery was realised. These were such people as the teaching staff, learners (other than nurses, who were recorded in this study), senior nursing and medical staff not actually part of the theatre team but there for other purposes, sometimes work-study people, and people such as the observer in this study. Although staff were asked about the effect of the observer's presence, it is felt that a record of the effect of the presence of any others would have made a useful contribution. One of the anecdotal comments refers to what one sister saw as her most nearly ideal list when there were no 'others' of any sort present.

The research design

It would have been more satisfactory to have been able to design a study that balanced objective theatre information with objective ward information, as was the case with the subjective information. This was recognised from the start as being a weakness but, in spite of this, the overrun/underrun time was identified as stressful in ward areas, and satisfaction was discovered to reflect at a significant level between ward and theatre areas.

Although the conclusions of this first research study into possible causes of additional stress in qualified nurses on operating days can only be presented as tentative, it is hoped that some of the significant stress measurements associated with management elements in the work environment may provide useful and usable indicators to those with responsibility for recruiting, retaining and managing nurses in these acute specialised areas.

Appendix I

From: The Department of Nursing, University of Manchester

Date

Name

Post Title

Hospital

Town

County

Dear

At present I am studying at University of Manchester for the degree of Master of Science (Nursing). I am planning to study stress influences on qualified nursing staff in the wards and theatres on operating days. I would like to undertake part of my study at (   ) hospital, as I (trained/worked) there between (19   and 19   ) and hope that this will be possible. My study will involve an interview with the senior nurse in the ward or theatre, and the recording of some environmental and organisational elements within the operating theatre.

I enclose a stamped, addressed envelope for your reply.

Yours sincerely,

Charmian Astbury

Appendix II

Check-list

- Time allowed for session
- Time used for session
- Number of operations per session
- Additions (i) at end of list, (ii) during list
- Control of premedication
- Control of cases
- Patient crisis
- Number of nursing staff
- Number of theatre-experienced nursing staff
- On-call staff
- Staff who stay late
- Meal-break problems

Critical incident form

Satisfying incidents						Score	Total	Code
	5	4	3	2	1			
	5	4	3	2	1			
	5	4	3	2	1			

Stressful incidents						Score	Total	Code
	5	4	3	2	1			
	5	4	3	2	1			
	5	4	3	2	1			

Date:
a.m. or p.m.:
Theatre or ward:
Number of cases:

Note:
5 = extremely satisfying/stressful
4 = very satisfying/stressful
3 = satisfying/stressful
2 = worth mention
1 = just worth mention

Appendix III

RESEARCH INSTRUMENT (MAIN STUDY)

A. Objective variables (theatres)

Survey number
```
        1    2
      ┌────┬────┐
      │    │    │
      └────┴────┘
```

Hospital
```
             3
           ┌────┐
           │    │
           └────┘
```

Theatre
```
             4
           ┌────┐
           │    │
           └────┘
```

Session   a.m. = 1, p.m. = 2, all-day = 3
```
             5
           ┌────┐
           │    │
           └────┘
```

Time allowed (hours and minutes)
```
      6    7    8
    ┌────┬────┬────┐
    │    │    │    │
    └────┴────┴────┘
```

Time taken (hours and minutes)
```
      9   10   11
    ┌────┬────┬────┐
    │    │    │    │
    └────┴────┴────┘
```

Delayed start (hours and minutes)
```
     12   13   14
    ┌────┬────┬────┐
    │    │    │    │
    └────┴────┴────┘
```

Number of operations
```
     15   16
    ┌────┬────┐
    │    │    │
    └────┴────┘
```

Number and type of operations
```
       17   18
     ┌────┬────┐
     │    │    │
     ├────┼────┤  19, 20
     │    │    │
     ├────┼────┤  21, 22
     │    │    │
     └────┴────┘
```

minor   1

intermediate   2

major   3

Control of premedication time
    anaesthetist = 1, theatre sister = 2, ward = 3
```
       23
     ┌────┐
     │    │
     └────┘
```

Control of operation time
  anaesthetist = 1, theatre sister = 2,
                    ward = 3

24

Alterations to list   yes = 1, no = 2

25

  additions   yes = 1, no = 2

26

  cancellations   yes = 1, no = 2

27

  order change   yes = 1, no = 2

28

  inaccuracies   yes = 1, no = 2

29

  uncommunicated changes
                    yes = 1, no = 2

30

Number of alterations

31   32

Morning list delivered previous
  afternoon
        yes = 1, no = 2, not applicable = 0

33

Afternoon list delivered previous
  afternoon
        yes = 1, no = 2, not applicable = 0

34

List typed   yes = 1, no = 2

35

Patient crisis   yes = 1, no = 2

36

TSSU   yes = 1, no = 2

37

Recovery room   yes = 1, no = 2

38

Receptionist/reception area
                    yes = 1, no = 2

39

Theatre temperature (°C)

40   41

Theatre humidity
  high = 1, normal = 2, low = 3

42

Theatre temperature perceived by staff as

        hot = 1, pleasant = 2, cold = 3

43

Window (outlook with horizon)

        yes = 1, no = 2

44

Type of theatre

45

        single = 1, twin = 2, multi-suite = 3

Staff shared between theatres

        yes = 1, no = 2, not applicable = 0

46

Standard counting/recording procedure

swabs	yes = 1, no = 2
needles	yes = 1, no = 2
instruments	yes = 1, no = 1

47

48

49

Number of qualified staff

50 51

Number of theatre-experienced qualified staff

52 53

Seniority of nurse in charge

        sister = 1, S/N = 2, SEN = 3

54

Number of learner nurses

55 56

Learners significant part of workforce

        yes = 1, no = 2, not applicable = 0

57

Number of nursing auxiliaries

58 59

'On-call' staff

        yes = 1, no = 2, not applicable = 0

60

Staff expected to stay late yes = 1, no = 2

61
[ ]

Meal breaks
   missed = 1, interrupted = 2,
                        taken properly = 3

62
[ ]

Anything observed that might indicate
stress (state observation)
                        yes = 1, no = 2

63
[ ]

80
[1]

B. Subjective variables (theatres and wards)

Survey number

1   2
[|]

Hospital

3
[ ]

Theatre

4
[ ]

Session   a.m. = 1, p.m. = 2, all day = 3

5
[ ]

1. Theatre
Satisfying incidents
   patient-centred

   staff-centred

   administration-centred

6
[   ]
7
8

Intensity (5 = high, 1 = low)
   patient-centred
   staff-centred
   adminstration-centred

9   10
[|]
11
13

Stressful incidents

   patient-centred

   staff-centred

   administration-centred

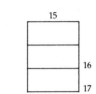

Intensity (5 = high, 1 = low)

   patient-centred

   staff-centred

   administration-centred

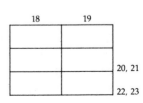

2. Ward

Satisfying incidents

   patient-centred

   staff-centred

   administration-centred

Intensity (5 = high, 1 = low)

   patient-centred

   staff-centred

   administration-centred

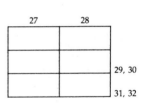

Stressful incidents

   patient-centred

   staff-centred

   administration-centred

Intensity (5 = high, 1 = low)

   patient-centred

   staff-centred

   administration-centred

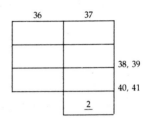

C. Critical incident sheet: theatre

Satisfying incidents
Patient-centred = P, staff-centred = S, administrative = A
Rating scale: high 5   4   3   2   1 low

P	x
S	x
A	x

Stressful incidents
Patient-centred = P, staff-centred = S, administration-centred = A
Rating scale: high 5   4   3   2   1 low

P	x
S	x
A	x

Anecdotal incidents

D. Critical incident sheet: ward

Satisfying incidents
Patient-centred = P, staff-centred = S, administrative = A
Rating scale: high 5   4   3   2   1

P	x
S	x
A	x

Stressful incidents

Patient-centred = P, staff-centred = S, administration-centred = A
Rating scale: high 5   4   3   2   1 low

P	x
S	x
A	x

Anecdotal incidents

Appendix IV

STUDY VARIABLES AND PRELIMINARY COMPUTER
ANALYSIS FINDINGS

Morning, afternoon and all-day session

The number and type of sessions observed broke down thus:

- morning sessions   45.0% of observed sessions   (n = 18)
- afternoon sessions 42.5% of observed sessions   (n = 17)
- all-day sessions   12.5% of observed sessions   (n = 5)

Significance
Theatre   Staff-centred satisfaction intensity/type of session was significant at $p < 0.03$.

Time allowed for each session

The time-allowed was $2 - 8\frac{1}{2}$ hours. The mode, the most commonly occurring time, was 3 hours and the mean, or average, was 4 hours.

There was no relationship between the time allowed for the session and the stress or satisfaction scores of the theatre and ward nursing staff in this study.

Time taken for each session

The range of time taken was $1\frac{1}{2} - 8\frac{1}{4}$ hours, 70% of the time taken during the observed session being 4 hours or less, with the mode at 3 hours and the mean at $4\frac{1}{4}$ hours.

There was no relationship between the time taken for the session and the stress or satisfaction scores of the theatre and ward nursing staff in this study.

Delayed start

Twenty-nine (72.5%) of all observed sessions started on time. The range of delay in this study was from 5 minutes to 1 hour 15 minutes, with 10% of the sessions starting half an hour late.

The delayed start was looked at in connection with alterations to the list, but no relationship was discovered. There was also no relationship between a delayed start and the stress or satisfaction scores of the theatre and ward nursing staff.

Overrun/underrun time

A time consideration was computed from variables 5 and 6 and variables 7 and 8, which was the difference between the time allowed and the time taken. This time was referrred to as the overrun/underrun time. The time range was 380 minutes (from -150 to $+230$ minutes).

- percentage of observed sessions overrunning   50.0%
- percentage of observed sessions underrunning   47.5%
- percentage of observed sessions finishing on time   2.5%

Significances
Theatre There was no significant relationship between the over-run/underrun time and the stress and satisfaction scores in staff.
Ward Significant correlations were found to exist between the overrun/underrun time and the stress scores of the nursing staff on the wards.
The results are:

- patient-centred incidents   number too small to use
- staff-centred incidents $p<0.005$
- administration-centred incidents $p<0.05$
- patient-centred intensity $p<0.037$
- staff-centred intensity $p<0.003$
- administration-centred intensity just failed to register at the
                                      significant level

Number of operations

The number of operations for the observed session ranged from $1-17$. The most commonly occurring number of operations for a routine session, the mode, was 4, which occurred in 27.5% of all lists.

There was no significant relationship observed between the number of operations on a list and the stress or satisfaction scores in theatre or ward nursing staff in this study.

Type of operation

The categorisation for the type of operation in this study was that of minor, intermediate or major.

- minor operations per observed list   range 0 – 13
- intermediate operations per observed list   range 0 – 9
- major operations per observed list   range 0 – 4

- 35.0% of lists had no minor surgery
- 25.0% of lists had no intermediate surgery
- 27.5% of lists had no major operations
- 32.5% of lists had one minor case
- 20.0% of lists had three intermediate operations
- 42.5% of lists had one major operation

There was no significant relationship discovered between the type of operation on a list and the stress or satisfaction scores in the theatre or ward nursing staff. A correlation between major operations and the overrun/underrun time just failed to register at the significant level.

Control of premedication time

The premedication time may be controlled by the anaesthetist, theatre sister or ward sister. The results in this study were:

- 95% of premedication times were controlled by the anaesthetist
- 5% of premedication times were controlled by the ward sister

There was no significant relationship discovered between the control of the premedication time and the stress or satisfaction scores of the theatre or ward nursing staff in this study.

Control of operation time

The time at which the next patient is sent for may be controlled by the anaesthetist, the theatre sister or the ward sister. The results of this study were that 100% of the control of the operation time was provided by the theatre sister.

There was no significant relationship between the control of the operation time and the stress or satisfaction scores of the the theatre or ward nursing staff in this study.

Alteration to the operating list

In this study 62.5% of operating lists were altered. This did not in itself register any significance in the stress or satisfaction scores of the nursing staff involved, but the breakdown in to types of alteration did.

Additions to the operating list

Thirty per cent of alterations were additions.

Significance
Theatre A significance was discovered to exist between the satisfaction scores of the theatre nursing staff patient-centred comments and additions to the list. This was significant at $p<0.005$.

Cancellations on the operating list

Forty per cent of all alterations were cancellations.

Significance
Theatre A significance was discovered to exist between the satisfaction scores of the theatre nursing staff in relation to the patient-centred incidents and cancellations to the list. The relationship patient-centred satisfaction incidents/cancellations was significant at $p<0.005$.

Order change

A change of order was noted in 20% of alterations to the list.

There was no significant relationship between the order of the operating list being changed and the stress or satisfaction scores of the theatre or ward nursing staff in this study.

Inaccuracies

Inaccuracies made up 2.5% of all alterations to the list.

Significance

Theatre A significant correlation was found to exist between inaccuracies and the staff-centred incident and intensity scores in relation to stress. The relationship staff-centred stress incidents/ inaccuracies was significant at $p<0.005$, and that of staff-centred stress intensity/inaccuracies significant at $p<0.013$.

Uncommunicated changes

Uncommunicated changes made up 7.5% of alterations to the operating list.

There was no significant relationship between the uncommunicated changes to the operating list and the stress or satisfaction scores of the theatre or ward nursing staff in this study.

Number of alterations

The number of alterations to an operating list in this study ranged from 0–6, with the mode being 1, and occurring 12 times.

There was no significant relationship discovered in this study between the number of alterations and the stress or satisfaction scores of the theatre or ward nursing staff.

Morning list delivered the previous afternoon

In all but one instance the morning list was delivered during the afternoon or late afternoon of the day prior to the morning operating session.

There was no significant correlation between the time of delivery of the morning list and the stress or satisfaction scores of the theatre or ward nursing staff in this study.

Afternoon list delivered the previous day

On six occasions the afternoon list was not delivered until the morning of the day of operation and in one hospital, every week, the list was not compiled until 2 hours before the afternoon session was due to start.

There was no significant relationship between the time of delivery of the afternoon list and the stress or satisfaction scores of the theatre or ward nursing staff in this study.

List typed

Of all operating lists, 47.5% were typed.

There was no significant relationship found to exist in this study between the list being typed and the stress or satisfaction scores of the theatre or ward nursing staff.

Patient crisis

A patient crisis occurred on 12.5% of all the observed operating lists.

Significance
Theatre   A significant correlation was found to exist between the experience of a patient-crisis in the operating theatre and the level of the stress intensity scores ($p<0.01$). (This data was subjected to analysis after all the categories of stress had been considered together. They were not considered independently as patient-centred, staff-centred or administration-centred stresses. This meant that a slightly higher figure was available for analysis in this pilot study. This particular probability, or significance, results from this slightly different approach.)

Presence of theatre sterile supply unit

In this study 65% of all observed sessions were supplied with sterile goods from a theatre sterile supply unit (TSSU).

Significance
Theatre   A significant relationship was found to exist in this study

between theatres that were not served by a TSSU and satisfaction scores, which was significant at the $p<0.01$ level.

Recovery room

All operating theatres in the study had the services of a recovery room.

There was no significant relationship found to exist between the presence of a recovery room and the stress and satisfaction scores of the theatre and ward nursing staff.

Receptionist/reception area

Ninety per cent of all operating theatres had a reception area, with or without a receptionist (that is, a non-nurse). There was no reception area in 10%.

There was no significant relationship found to exist between the presence of a reception area, either with or without a receptionist, and the stress or satisfaction scores of the theatre or ward nursing staff.

Theatre temperature

The range of temperature in the operating theatres was from 19°C–28°C, with 75% of the theatres having temperatures of 23°C or below. The mode was 22°C, occurring in 14 sessions.

There was no significant relationship found to exist between the temperature in the operating theatre and the stress or satisfaction scores of the theatre or ward nursing staff.

Theatre humidity

The humidity was recorded as high (above 60%), normal (approximately 55%) or low (below 50%).

- 50.0% of operating theatres registered humidity as high
- 47.5% of operating theatres registered humidity as normal
- 2.5% of operating theatres registered humidity as low

There was no significant correlation between the humidity and the stress or satisfaction scores of the theatre or ward nursing staff in this study.

Perception of temperature by staff

The variable was the perception of how the ambient temperature was experienced by the 'scrubbed' nursing staff. The classification was hot, pleasant or cold.

- 42.5% of staff perceived the temperature as hot
- 52.5% of staff perceived the temperature as pleasant
- 5.0% of staff perceived the temperature as cold

Significance
Theatre There was a significant correlation between the temperature perceived as hot and the stress scores in the operating theatre when the analysis used the non-categorised stress scores, that is, all incidents were described as 'stress' and not divided into the three categories. The relationship perception of temperature/stress incidents was highly significant at $p<0.001$, and that of perception of temperature/stress intensity significant at $p<0.01$.

Window (outlook with horizon)

In this study 57.5% of operating theatres were windowless.

Significance
Theatre A significant correlation was found to exist between stress scores in the operating theatre and the absence of windows. No windows/staff-centred stress incidents was significant at $p<0.0065$ and no windows/staff-centred intensity was significant at $p<0.01$.

Type of theatre

The classification in the study was single, twin or multi-suite theatre.

- 15% of observed sessions were in single theatres
- 50% of observed sessions were in twin theatres
- 35% of observed sessions were in multi-suite theatres

There was no significant relationship observed between the type of theatre and the stress or satisfaction scores of the theatre or ward nursing staff.

Staff shared between theatres

Of the staff in charge of the observed session, 65% stated that staff were taken from their teams to work in other theatre areas. There was no significant relationship between the sharing of staff between theatres and the stress or satisfaction scores of the theatre or ward nursing staff.

Standard counting/recording procedures

The staff in each observed session were seen to practise the procedure of their particular hospital.

There was no significant relationship found to exist between the carrying-out of standard procedures and the stress or satisfaction scores of the theatre or ward nursing staff.

Number of qualified staff

The number of qualified staff for each session was:

- 2 qualified nurses in 67.5% of observed sessions
- 3 qualified nurses in 27.5% of observed sessions
- 4 qualified nurses in 5.1% of observed sessions

Significance

Theatre A significant correlation was found to exist between the presence of qualified nursing staff and administration-centred incidents of satisfaction. Small number size precluded specific analysis in relation to numbers of staff. The relationship qualified nursing staff/administrative satisfaction incidents was significant at $p<0.05$.

Number of theatre-experienced qualified nursing staff

The number of qualified nursing staff with theatre experience present during each observed session was found to be:

- no such nurse present at 2.5% of sessions
- 1 such nurse present at 17.5% of sessions
- 2 such nurses present at 40.0% of sessions
- 3 such nurses present at 35.0% of sessions
- 4 such nurses present at 5.0% of sessions

Significance
Theatre A significant correlation was found to exist between the presence of theatre-experienced qualified staff and staff-centred stress ($p<0.03$). Small number size precluded specific analysis in relation to numbers of staff.

Seniority of nurse in charge

The seniority of the nurse in charge of each observed session was described by grade, that is, either sister, staff nurse or state enrolled nurse.

- 82.5% of observed sessions had a sister in charge
- 15.0% of observed sessions had a staff nurse in charge
- 2.5% of observed sessions had a state enrolled nurse in charge

No significant relationship was found to exist between the seniority of the nurse in charge and the stress or satisfaction scores of the theatre or ward nursing staff.

Number of learner nurses

The number of learner nurses present (student or pupil nurses) ranged from 0 – 4, 70% of the observed sessions having none or only one present. This was an area that looked as though a significant level for stress would emerge but, when the specific test for small group numbers was applied, this was found not to be the case.

There was no significant relationship between the number of learner nurses and the stress or satisfaction scores of the theatre or ward nursing staff.

Learners as a significant part of the work force

When learners were present, 96% of the time they were used as a significant part of the work force.

There was no significant relationship found to exist between the use of learners as a significant part of the work force and the stress or satisfaction scores of the theatre or ward nursing staff.

Number of nursing auxiliaries

The number of nursing auxiliaries present during each observed session was found to be:

- no auxiliaries present in 45.0% of all observed sessions
- 1 auxiliary present in 50.0% of all observed sessions
- 2 auxiliaries present in 5.0% of all observed sessions

There was no significant relationship found to exist between the number of nursing auxiliaries present and the stress or satisfaction scores of the theatre or ward nursing staff.

'On-call' staff

The classification used here was based on the answers 'yes', 'no' and 'not applicable'. Twenty-eight per cent of the staff to whom the question applied stated that they were expected to be 'on-call'.

There was no significant relationship between those who were expected to undertake 'on-call' duties and the stress or satisfaction scores of the theatre or ward nursing staff.

Staff who were expected to stay late

Of staff working in the theatres during the observed sessions, 87.5% were expected to stay late.

Significance
Theatre   It was discovered that there was a correlation between this percentage and certain satisfaction scores in the theatre staff. Expected to stay late/patient-centred satisfaction was significant at $p<0.03$, and expected to stay late/administration-centred satisfaction was significant at $p<0.04$.

Meal breaks

The meal break variable was divided into those missed (2.5%), those interrupted (25%) and those taken properly (72.5%).

There was no significant relationship discovered between these categories and stress or satisfaction scores, but a significant correlation was found to exist with meal breaks as such and the stress scores of nursing staff in the theatre.

Significance

Theatre It was discovered that there was a correlation between stress scores of theatre nursing staff and meal breaks, with relationships significant as follows:

- patient-centred stress incidents/meal breaks significant at $p<0.007$
- patient-centred stress intensity/meal breaks significant at $p<0.004$
- administration-centred incidents/meal breaks significant at $p<0.04$

Observations that might indicate stress

During 57.5% of the observed sessions there appeared to be visible signs of stress in staff. There was a significant correlation between observed stress and staff stress incidents and intensity.

Significance

Theatre The relationship staff-centred stress incidents/observed stress was significant at $p<0.034$, while that of staff-centred stress intensity/observed stress was significant at $p<0.036$.

Two additional analyses were conducted.
1. *Reflection of stress/satisfaction scores* The data was analysed in order to discover whether or not stress or satisfaction were reflected between the scores of the nurses in the theatres and the scores of the nurses on the wards. No significant correlation was found in relation to the stress scores, but one did appear in relation to satisfaction.

- Patient-centred intensity of experience for satisfaction in the operating theatres correlated with patient-centred intensity of experience for satisfaction in the wards. This was significant at $p<0.032$.
- Patient-centred intensity of experience for satisfaction in the operating theatres correlated with administration-centred intensity of experience of satisfaction in the wards. This was significant at $p<0.017$.

2. *Correlation between high stress and low satisfaction* The data was analysed in order to ascertain whether or not a correlation would be

found to exist between high scores for stress and low scores for satisfaction in the theatres and in the wards. A significant correlation was found to exist in the scores of the theatre nursing staff.

- satisfaction score (incidents) low/stress score (incidents) high at $p<0.007$
- satisfaction score (incidents) low/stress (intensity) high at $p<0.008$
- satisfaction score (intensity) low/stress score (incidents) high at $p<0.021$
- satisfaction score (intensity) low/stress score (intensity) high at $p<0.034$

This particular analysis further indicated that the satisfaction scores for intensity and incidents, and the stress scores for incidents and intensity for both the ward and theatre nursing staffs, related within each particular group at the highly significant level of $p<0.001$.

Appendix V

SELECTION OF NURSING STAFF INTERVIEW COMMENTS

Patient-centred comments and intensity scores: satisfaction

Theatre staff

'There was time to feel confident and secure with the patients today' (4)

'There was time to feel satisfied with what one was able to do for the patients' (4)

'It's satisfying to get these little jobs done for the patients' (3)

'Getting the patients through all right' (3)

Ward staff

'Being able to ensure each patient's comfort' (4)

'Going home shattered after these busy lists, but with a marvellous feeling that all the patients have been treated safely' (5)

'They've started to use a new bowel prep – still unpleasant for them, but much better than the old one, far less exhausting' (5)

'Now that most premeds on this ward are oral, it doesn't matter so much what they do to the list' (4)

Patient-centred comments and intensity scores: stress

Theatre staff

'The additional patient being cancelled' (2)

'The rather frail patient' (3)

'The cancellation of the last patient – and she's one of our theatre staff' (3)

'This elderly patient, living alone and a day case – he'd had breakfast' (3)

Ward staff
   'List changes like today's make the patients anxious – they know what order they should be going in' (4)
   'These sorts of patient who are becoming long-stay – not well enough for surgery and not well enough for transfer' (4)
   'The patients have moved round this ward twice today, in the one shift. They've decided to open the closed beds. It's been impossible' (5)
   'These two old ladies have been starved for two days, but at last they've had a drip put up' (5)

Staff-centred comments and intensity scores: satisfaction

Theatre staff
   'Sufficient staff of right calibre' (5)
   'Mix of staff enabled me to teach, and give experience to learners' (4)
   'Surgeons agreeable' (4)
   'Good team today, everyone worked together' (3)

Ward staff
   'Sufficient staff to look after the patients' (4)
   'Enough staff of the right calibre – and a ward clerk' (4)
   'Very even list today, and sufficient staff and not many learners' (3)
   'Today's been fine – no-one's been taken away' (3)

Staff-centred comments and intensity scores: stress

Theatre staff
   'Too many learners, not enough trained staff, and this is a long, quick list' (4)
   'This surgeon likes noise at a minimum, and he always finds the theatre too hot' (2)
   'The rush and pressure at the lunchtime changeover' (4)
   'Today we had inexperienced staff, brand new staff and the sister and surgeon who don't like each other' (4)

Ward staff
'All the additional work concerning the cancellation, phoning relatives and all the rest of it' (5)
'The pressure from the doctors – always wanting you to do things for them' (4)
'The new staff and the list changes' (5)
'Biggest problem is the surgeon – Mondays are frightful. The patients are admitted, but no-one knows who's for theatre until after the morning round' (5)

Administration-centred comments and intensity scores: satisfaction

Theatre staff
'Management of the equipment and instruments fine today, no hold-ups' (4)
'No time pressures' (4)
'No problem with equipment, even though there's only the one cystoscope he likes to use' (3)
'Everything went smoothly' (3)

Ward staff
'This highly organised routine for these busy op days – it makes you feel you've achieved something' (5)
'We've a ward clerk, no admin burdens whatsoever' (4)
'We've only two consultants and their two house officers to fit in' (4)
'We got the rounds in before the list started. That's what I like' (3)

Administration-centred comments and intensity scores: stress

Theatre staff
'The supply of instruments did not keep up with the patients' (4)
'The addition being cancelled' (3)
'I don't like having to tackle this sort of list when I've been up in the night. I wasn't on call as such, but they had two teams out finishing the day's surgery, and had to call us in for the emergencies' (5)

'The electrician; I didn't know what he was meant to do. No-one tells me anything' (4)

Ward staff
'The beds – having to get the patients home, transferring them, borrowing beds from other wards' (4)
'The phones ringing all at once' (5)
'The porter came for the wrong patient' (5)
'The porter arrived before the first patient was even ready' (4)

Selection of Anecdotal Comments

'Every week lists over overbooked, surgeons arrive late and then teach on every patient. They forget at five that we've been here since eight' (theatre stress)
'Biggest problem is always lack of beds – last week we had twelve outliers' (ward stress)
'Porter turned up yesterday at 8.25 a.m. for a patient who was fourth on a list that was due to start at 8.15 a.m. (ward stress)
'In the 7 weeks we've been in this new theatre, only 3 out of the 39 staff have not been off sick – that's me [the nursing officer] and two of the ODAs' (theatre stress)
'The all-day list is a stress. The late mix of staff is nearly always very poor – one trained, one auxiliary and a learner' (ward stress)
'The best list we've had for ages was six weeks ago – there were no learners of any sort whatsoever, no nurses, no medics, no trainee ODAs, just ourselves' (theatre stress)

The anecdotal comments were not rated for intensity of perception. The criterion for inclusion in this selection of comments was the general representativeness of the comment made. There were far more experiences recalled that were stress experiences. It is interesting to compare the recalled experiences with the here-and-now experiences of the observed routine sessions in which satisfaction was the predominant experience.

Appendix VI

STATISTICAL TESTS FOR NON-PARAMETRIC DATA

These tests were all applied in the study. For further information see Siegel, 1956.

Chi-square test

Should the data consist of frequencies in discrete categories, the chi-squared test may be used to determine the difference between two or more independent groups.

Fisher's exact probability test

This test should be applied when two independent samples are small in size. It is used when the scores from two independent samples fall into one or other of two mutually exclusive classes.

Kruskal-Wallis one-way anova

This test is used where at least an ordinal measurement has been achieved. It can be used to decide whether independent samples are from different populations. It is a generalised version of the Mann-Whitney U test, and is based on the assignment of ranks to the scores of the various groups.

Mann-Whitney U test

This test may be used to establish whether two independent groups have been drawn from the same population where at least an ordinal measurement has been achieved.

Spearman correlation coefficient

This is a statistical procedure used where ordinal ranking has been achieved. A correlation coefficient summarises the magnitude of the relationship between variables.

Wilcoxon rank sum test

This is a procedure for testing the difference between samples.

References

Annadale-Steiner D (1979) Unhappiness in the nurse who expected more. *Nursing Mirror*, 149(22): 34–36.

Archer S E, Kelly C D and Bisch S A (1984) *Implementing Change in Communities*. Toronto: C V Mosby.

Aries J (1981) The 37½-hour working week for nurses, its implementation and implications in the operating department. *NAT News*, February: 17–26.

Barr A (1967) *Measure of Nursing Care*. Report No. 9. Oxford Regional Hospital Board.

Baxter B (1971) The nurse in the operating room complex. *Nursing Times*, **67(38)**: 1190.

Boore J R P (1978) *Prescription for Recovery*. RCN Research Series. London: Royal College of Nursing.

Bosanquet N (1974) Theatre nurses and Whitehall. *Nursing Times*, **70(43)**: 1667–1668.

Brett H (1976) Five years on II. *Nursing Times*, **72(42)**, Theatre Nursing Supplement: 5.

Brett H (1978) 'Did we stick to the brief? *Nursing Times*, **74(42)**: 1717–1718.

Brigden R J (1974) *Operating Theatre Technique*, 3rd edn. Edinburgh: Churchill Livingstone.

Campbell M (1979) *Theatre Routine*, 2nd edn. London: Heinemann Medical Books.

Carr A (1978) Cost-effective nursing. *Nursing Times*, **74(22)**: 906–907.

Charnley J (1970) Operating theatre ventilation. *Lancet* **i**: 1053–1054.

Clark J M and Hockey L (1979) *Research for Nursing*. Aylesbury: HM and M Publishers.

Claus K E and Bailey J T (1977) *Power and Influence in Health Care*. St Louis: C V Mosby.

Coghill N F, Revans R W, Ulyatt F M and Ulyatt K W (1970) A Study of Consultants. *Lancet*, **ii**: 305–307.

Coghill N F (1972) Letters to Editor: Management in Health Services. *Lancet*, **ii**: 1063–1064.

Coleman V (1978) *Stress Control*. London: Maurice Temple Smith.

The Committee on Nursing (1972) Chairman: Asa Briggs. *Report presented to Parliament by the Secretary of State for Social Services, the Secretary of State for Scotland and the Secretary of State for Wales by Command of Her Majesty.* London: HMSO.

Cox M P (1974) A layman looks at Lewin. *Nursing Times,* **70 (15)**: 560–561.

Craig B J (1978) Team leader concept implemented in the OR. *AORN Journal,* **28(4)**: 726–732.

Cranfield A B (1972) *Theatre Nurses' Handbook.* London: Butterworths.

Davies J (1972) *A Study of Hospital Management Training.* Centre for Business Research in association with Manchester Business School, University of Manchester.

Department of Health and Social Security, Welsh Office, Central Health Services Council (1970) Chairman: Walpole Lewin, FRCS. *The Organisation and Staffing of Operating Departments.* London: HMSO.

Department of Health and Social Security (1974) Chairman: The Right Honourable the Earl of Halsbury, FRS. *Report of the Committee of Inquiry into Pay and Related Conditions of Service of Nurses and Midwives.* London: HMSO.

Diers D (1979) *Research in Nursing Practice.* Philadelphia: J B Lippincott.

Dixon E P (1976) *An Introduction to the Operating Theatre.* Edinburgh: Churchill Livingstone.

Dixon E P (1978) The legal aspects of surgery. *NAT News,* November: 12–20.

Downie R S and Calman K C (1987) *Healthy Respect. Ethics in Health Care.* London: Faber and Faber.

Drucker P (1967) *The Effective Executive.* London: Pan Books, in association with William Heinemann.

Dudley H A (1976) Operative ergonomics. *Nursing Mirror,* **143(18)**: 53–54.

Duffey I M and Worthington J M (1980) Effects of changes made in operating lists. Unpublished paper presented to colleagues at Manchester Royal Infirmary.

Elliott J (1966) Change partners. *Lancet,* **ii**: 1068–1070.

Fish E J (1974) Theatre nurse training course. *Nursing Times,* **70(43)**: 1658–1660.

Flanagan J C (1954) The critical incident technique. *Psychological Bulletin* **51(4)**: 327–357.

Freeman D M (1976) *Operating Theatre Suites Staff Workload Comparison*. Unpublished paper, Southampton General Hospital.

Gatley M S (1981) Mental health aspects of occupational health. *The Royal Society of Health Journal*, **101(4)**: 141 – 147.

Gebhard P H (1978) Stressor aspects of societal attitudes to sex roles and relationships. In: *Society, Stress and Disease*, vol.3, ed. Levi L. Oxford: Oxford University Press.

Goodman J A (1978) Institutionalised sexism as a social constraint in male/female interaction. In: *Society, Stress and Disease*, vol 3 ed. Levi L. Oxford: Oxford University Press.

Great Britain Central Health Services Council and Scottish Health Services Council (1968). Chairman: Sir Ronald Tunbridge. *Care of the Health of Hospital Staff* London: HMSO.

Greaves D (1974) Operating in 'best buy' Bury St Edmunds. *Nursing Times*, **70(43)**: 1664 – 1666.

Gruendemann B J (1975) The impact of surgery on body image. *Nursing Clinics of North America*, **10(4)**: 49. Philadelphia: W B Saunders.

Hamilton-Smith S (1972) *Nil by Mouth?* RCN Research Series. London: Royal College of Nursing.

Handy C B (1985) *Understanding organisations*, 3rd edn. Harmondsworth: Penguin Books.

Hassell D (1971) Theatre staffing – a need for change. *Nursing Times*, Occasional Papers, **67(4)**: 13 – 15.

Hay D and Oken D (1972) The psychological stresses of intensive care unit nursing. *Psychosomatic Medicine*, **34(2)**: 109 – 118.

Hayward J (1975) *Information – A Prescription Against Pain*. RCN Research Series. London: Royal College of Nursing.

Heath J and Law G M (1982) *Nursing Process – What is it?* Sheffield: NHS Learning Resources Unit.

Henderson V (1966) *The Nature of Nursing*. London: Collier Macmillan.

Herzberg F (1966) The motivation-hygiene theory. In: *Management and Motivation*, eds. Vroom V H and Deci E L (1970). Harmondsworth: Penguin Modern Management Classics.

Hillier S (1980) Stress, strain and smoking. *Nursing Mirror*, **152(7)**: 26 – 27.

Hindle A (1970) *A Simulation Approach to Surgical Scheduling*. Department of Operational Research, University of Lancaster.

Hingley P, Cooper C and Harris P (1986) *Stress in Nurse Managers*. London: Kings Fund Centre.

Hockey L (1976) *Women in Nursing.* Sevenoaks: Hodder and Stoughton.

Hoeller M L (1974) *Surgical Technology: Basis for Clinical Practice,* 3rd edn. St Louis: C V Mosby.

Holesclaw P A (1965) Nursing in high emotional risk areas. *Nursing Forum,* **4(4)**: 36 – 45.

Howorth F H (1981) What's in the air of the operating theatre? *NAT News,* February: 10 – 19.

Hughes B C (1981) The use of modular operating theatres for modern surgery. *The Royal Society of Health Journal,* **101(4)**: 136 – 137.

Hulme M (1973) Nursing in the operating theatre. *Nursing Mirror,* **137**: 30 – 32.

Hunter B (1972) *The Administration of Hospital Wards: Factors Influencing Lengths of Stay in Hospital.* Manchester: Manchester University Press.

Janis I L (1958) *Psychological Stress.* New York, San Francisco, London: Academic Press.

Kinston W (1987) *Stronger Nursing Organisation: A Working Paper for General Managers and Nursing Managers.* A Health Services Centre Working Paper, Brunel Institute of Organisation and Social Studies, Brunel University.

Kogan H, Cang S, Dixon H and Tolliday H (1971) *Working Relationships with the British Hospital Service.* London: Bookstall Publications.

Lamont S J (1977) Thermal comfort for theatre personnel during surgical operations. *NAT News,* February: 10 – 14.

Lazarus R S (1964) *Personality and Adjustment,* 2nd edn. Englewood Cliffs, New Jersey: Prentice-Hall.

Leatt P and Schneck R (1980) Differences in stress perceived by head nurses across nursing operations. *Journal of Advanced Nursing,* **5**: 31 – 44.

Lewin W (1978) The organisation and staffing of operating departments. *Nursing Times,* **74(42)**: 1711 – 1712.

Likert R (1961) The effects of measurements on management practices. In: *Management and Motivation,* eds. Vroom V H and Deci E L (1970). Harmondsworth: Penguin Books.

Lunn J A (1975) *The Health of Staff in Hospital.* London: Heinemann Medical Books.

Maggs C (1981) Control mechanisms and the 'new nurses' 1881 – 1914. *Nursing Times,* Occasional Papers, **77(36)**: 97 – 100.

Maslow A H (1943) A theory of human motivation. In: *Management and Motivation*, eds. Vroom V H and Deci E L (1970). London: Penguin Books.

Maslow A H (1970) *Motivation and Personality*, 2nd edn. New York and London: Harper and Row.

Matthias M (1973) The operating department team. *Nursing Times*, **69(38)**: 1232–1233.

McFarlane J K (1978) *Nursing: the State of the Art*. Proceedings of the *Nursing Mirror* First International Cancer Nursing Care Conference. London: *Nursing Mirror*.

McGregor D M (1957) The human side of enterprise. In: *Management and Motivation*. eds. Vroom V H and Deci E L (1970). Harmondsworth: Penguin Books.

Medical Defence Union and Royal College of Nursing Joint Memorandum (1978a) *Safeguards against the Wrong Operations* London: The Medical Defence Union and The Royal College of Nursing.

Medical Defence Union and Royal College of Nursing Joint Memorandum (1978b) *Safeguards against Failure to Remove Swabs and Instruments from Patients*. London: The Medical Defence Union and The Royal College of Nursing.

Melia K H (1977) The intensive care unit – a stress situation. *Nursing Times*, Occasional Papers, **73(5)**: 17–20.

Menzies I E P (1970) *The Functioning of Social Systems as a Defence against Anxiety*. London: Centre for Applied Social Research, The Tavistock Institute of Human Relations.

Munday A (1973) *Physiological Measures of Anxiety in Hospital Patients*. RCN Research Series. London: Royal College of Nursing.

Murphy F, Bentley S, Ellis B W and Dudley H (1977) Sleep deprivation in patients undergoing operations: a factor in the stress of surgery. *British Medical Journal*, **ii**: 1521–1522.

National Audit Office (1987) *Use of Operating Theatres in the National Health Service*. Report by the Comptroller and Auditor General. London: HMSO.

Nichols K, Springford V and Searle J (1981) An investigation of distress and discontent in various types of nursing. *Journal of Advanced Nursing*, **6**: 311–318.

Nolan M G (1975) Foreword: Symposium on perspectives in operating room nursing. *Nursing Clinics of North America*, **10(4)**: 613–686. Philadelphia: W B Saunders.

Norris W and Campbell D (1975) *A Nurse's Guide to Anaesthetics, Resuscitation and Intensive Care*, 6th edn. Edinburgh: Churchill Livingstone.

Nursing Times (1979) Nurse, could you care more? *Nursing Times*, **75(13)**: 1610.

O'Connor V (1971) A world of its own: the operating department. *Nursing Times*, **67(42)**: 1307–1309.

Pembrey S (1980) *The Ward Sister – Key to Nursing*. RCN Research Series. London: Royal College of Nursing.

Perry E L (1978) *Ward Management and Teaching*. London: Baillière Tindall.

Peters T J and Waterman R M Jnr (1982) *In Search of Excellence*. New York: Harper and Row.

Phillips D (1981) *Do It Yourself Social Surveys: A Handbook for Beginners*. London: The Polytechnic of North London.

Phillips J (1980) Big is best? A study into the optimum size of multi-suite operating departments. *NAT News*, May: 7–14.

Polit D and Hungler B (1978) *Nursing Research: Principles and Practice*. Philadelphia: J B Lippincott.

Pollitt J (1977) Symptoms of stress I. Types of stress and types of people. *Nursing Mirror* **144(24)**: 13–14.

Rait A (1976) After Lewin. *Nursing Times*, **72(6)**: 206.

Revans R W (1964) *Standards for Morale*. Published for the Nuffield Provincial Hospitals Trust by the Oxford University Press, London, New York and Toronto.

Revans R W (1971) Introduction. In: *Changing Hospitals*. A report on the Hospital Internal Communications Project, eds. Weiland G F and Leigh C. London: Tavistock Publications.

Revans R W (1972) Introduction. In: *Hospitals: Communication, Choice and Change*, ed. Revans R W. London: Tavistock Publications.

Revans R W (1976) *Action Learning in Hospitals*. London: McGraw-Hill.

Rhys-Hearn (1972) How many high care patients? II. *Nursing Times*, **68(17)**: 504–505.

Robson M (1986) *The Journey to Excellence*. Chichester: John Wiley and Sons.

Roper N, Logan W W and Tierney A J (1980) *The Elements of Nursing*. Edinburgh: Churchill Livingstone.

Ross T (1977) Theatre horizons, theatre people. *Nursing Mirror*, **145(14)**, Special Theatre Supplement: iii–x.

Rowbottom R (1973) *Hospital Organisation*. London: Heinemann.

Rowntree D (1981) *Statistics without Tears*. Harmondsworth: Penguin Books.

Royal College of Nursing (1968) *The Implementation of a Hospital Occupational Health Service*. London: Royal College of Nursing.

Royal College of Nursing (1978) *Counselling in Nursing*. The report of a working party held under the auspices of The RCN Institute of Advanced Nursing Education. London: Royal College of Nursing.

Selye H (1965) The stress of life. New focal points for understanding accidents. *Nursing Forum,* **4(1)**: 29 – 38.

Selye H (1978) *The Stress of Life*, 2nd edn. (revised). New York: McGraw-Hill.

Shepherd B J (1976) Training of learners in the theatre unit. *Nursing Times,* **72(42)**, Theatre Nursing Supplement: 7 – 10.

Siegel S (1956) *Non-parametric statistics for the behavioural sciences*. New York, London: McGraw-Hill Kogakusha Ltd.

Stephens D S B and Boaler J (1977) The nurse's role in immediate post-operative care. *Nursing Mirror,* **145(13)**: 20 – 23.

Sweeney M A and Olivieri P (1981) An introduction to nursing research. Research, Measurement and Computers in Nursing. Philadelphia: J B Lippincott.

Tobin H M (1974) *The Process of Staff Development*. St Louis: C V Mosby.

Toffler A (1970) *Future Shock*. London: Pan Books.

Toynbee A (1966) *A Study of History*. Oxford: Oxford University Press.

Treece E W and Treece J W (1977) *Elements of Research in Nursing*. St Louis: C V Mosby.

Wallace M (1978) Living with stress. *Nursing Times,* **74(11)**: 457 – 458.

White R W (1976) Strategies of adaptation. In: *Human Adaptations: Coping with Life Crises*, ed. Moos R. Lexington, Mass., Toronto: D. C. Heath.

Willingham J (1971) *Operating Theatre Techniques*. London: Heinemann Medical.

Wilson-Barnett J (1979) *Stress in Hospital: Patients' Psychological Reactions to Illness and Health Care*. Edinburgh: Churchill Livingstone.

Woolstone A S (1978) Stress – a call for a humane approach. *Nursing Times,* **74(14)**: 599 – 600.